RIP7

Field's

Lower Limb Anatomy, Palpation and Surface Markings

For Elsevier:

Commissioning Editor: Robert Edwards
Development Editor: Barbara Simmons
Production Manager: Susan Stuart
Project Management and Typesetting: Helius
Design: Andrew Chapman
Illustrator: Derek Field
Cover Design: Kneath Associates

Field's

Lower Limb Anatomy, Palpation and Surface Markings

Derek Field Grad Dip Phys, FCSP, Dip TP
Former Vice Principal , North London School of Physiotherapy, City University, London

Jane Owen Hutchinson MA(ED), MCSP, SRP, Dip TP
Manager, Physiotherapy Support Service, Royal National Institute of the Blind, London

Edited with a Foreword by Anthony Redmond

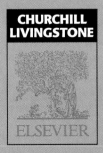

EDINGBURGH LONDON NEW YORK OXFORD PHILADELPHIA ST LOUIS SYDNEY TORONTO 2008

CHURCHILL
LIVINGSTONE
ELSEVIER

An imprint of Elsevier Limited

ISBN: 978 0 7020 3018 5

British Library Cataloguing in Publication Data
A catalogue record for this book is available from the British Library.

Library of Congress Cataloging in Publication Data
A catalog record for this book is available from the Library of Congress.

ELSEVIER your source for books, journals and multimedia in the health sciences
www.elsevierhealth.com

Working together to grow
libraries in developing countries

www.elsevier.com | www.bookaid.org | www.sabre.org

ELSEVIER   BOOK AID International   Sabre Foundation

The publisher's policy is to use paper manufactured from sustainable forests

Printed in China.

Contents

Foreword   vii

1. Palpation: principles and practice   1

Definitions and concepts   2
   Palpation: definitions   2
   General characteristics of palpation   2
Touch   2
   General characteristics   2
   The physiology of touch   3
   The social significance of touch   4
   Touch and clinical practice   5
Effects of palpation on the patient   6
   Patient and person   6
   The consultation process   7
Techniques of palpation   8
Improving the art of palpation   9
Care of the hands   10
Palpation of different tissues   10
Summary   12

2. Bones   15

The lumbar spine and pelvis   16
   The thoracic outlet   16
   The pelvic girdle   17
   The lumbar vertebrae   18
   The sacrum   18
   The coccyx   19
The hip region   20
The knee region   24
   Anterior aspect   25
   Medial aspect   26
   Lateral aspect   28
   Posterior aspect   30
The ankle region   32
   The lower end of the tibia   32
   The lower end of the fibula   32
   The talus   32
   The calcaneus   33
The calcaneous   34
The foot   36
   Dorsal aspect   36
   Plantar aspect   38
Self-assessment questions   40

3. Joints   57

The lumbar spine   58
The pelvis   62
The pubic symphysis   62

The sacroiliac joint   64
The hip joint   66
The knee joint   68
The tibiofibular union   72
   The superior tibiofibular joint   72
   The inferior tibiofibular joint   73
The ankle joint   74
The foot   78
   The talocalcaneal (subtalar) joint   78
   The talocalcaneonavicular joint   82
   The calcaneocuboid joint   84
   The cuboideonavicular joint   85
   The midtarsal joint   85
   The cuneonavicular and intercuneiform joints   86
   The tarsometatarsal joints   87
   The intermetatarsal joints   88
   The metatarsophalangeal joints   90
   The interphalangeal joints   92
Self-assessment questions   94

4. Muscles   109

The lateral and anterior aspect of the hip   110
   Gluteus medius, gluteus minimus and
     tensor fasciae latae   110
   Iliopsoas and pectineus   111
The posterior aspect of the hip and thigh   112
   Gluteus maximus   112
   The hamstrings   112
The anterior and medial aspects of the thigh   114
   The adductors and quadriceps femoris   114
   Sartorius   115
The anterior and lateral aspects of the lower
leg and foot   116
   Tibialis anterior   116
   Extensor hallucis longus   116
   Extensor digitorum longus   116
   Peroneus tertius   117
   Extensor digitorum brevis   117
The posterior and plantar aspects of the lower
leg and foot   118
   Popliteus   118
   Triceps surae (calf)   118
   Plantar muscles   120
Self-assessment questions   122

5. Nerves   133

Sciatic nerve and its derivatives   134
Self-assessment questions   136

6. Arteries   139

Femoral artery   140
Anterior and posterior tibial arteries   141
Self-assessment questions   142

7. Veins   145

The deep veins   146
The superficial veins   146

The great (long) saphenous vein   146
The small (short) saphenous vein   147
Self-assessment questions   148

References and further reading   *151*
Index   *153*

Foreword

The original *Anatomy, Palpation and Surface Markings* by Derek Field and Jane Owen Hutchinson was first published in 1994 and has since become one of the most successful and best loved practical anatomy texts. The main title is now in its fourth edition and its combination of meaningful clinical anatomy, clear photographs, helpful diagrams and self-assessment sections is tried and tested.

This new spin-off version focuses on the lower limb, an often neglected area of anatomy study. Although based on the parent text, it has been specifically reworked for students of lower limb structure and function.

In departments such as my own, with its mix of clinicians, researchers and trainees, there is always a need and an appetite for a better understanding of leg and foot anatomy. The aim of this version of Field's is to provide for the reader with an interest in the lower limb, both an impetus to think about leg and foot anatomy from a clinical perspective and an anatomy primer of real practical worth.

Lower Limb Anatomy, Palpation and Surface Markings will be of use to: lower limb specialists, such as podiatrists in training; other therapists and coaches with a contextual interest in the lower limb; junior doctors, for whom the detail of lower limb anatomy may have been lost in the milieu of whole body anatomy and biological sciences that often overwhelm the first years of study; and, of course, established clinicians in search of an anatomy refresher that has real practical application in their day-to-day practice.

From the outset, the approach in the Field's texts has been to help develop an appreciation of applied anatomy through direct palpation and the development of an understanding of the relationship between deep structures and the surface. In short, the ability to visualize deep anatomical structures through the skin – a very valuable clinical skill.

This skill is introduced explicitly in the opening chapter, which covers the characteristics of palpation and introduces relevant techniques. The rest of the book is set out in a consistent structure, with bones, joints, muscles and the neurovascular anatomy each covered in separate chapters. The individual chapters adopt a proximal to distal progression, starting with the lower back and pelvis and ending with the feet.

Pages are generously adorned with large, full-colour, labelled photographs that set out clearly the surface anatomy, highlighting anatomical landmarks and providing a visual anchor for clinical interpretation. The lower limb title continues the established and successful format of previous editions, pairing the clinical photographs with similarly labelled line drawings on facing pages. This approach helps the reader to contextualize the deep anatomy relative to the surface findings and provides strong graphical reinforcement. The supporting text provides the necessary anatomical detail along with clear instructions to aid the reader in accurately palpating the relevant structures. Finally, each chapter finishes with a revision and self-assessment section, cross-referenced to the relevant page in the main text, which will help the motivated reader to consolidate their knowledge. Where specific answers may not be found in the text itself, the question is followed by a sign (fr), which indicates that further reading from other texts is required.

This is a book that brings lower limb anatomy to life, and it is our hope that students of leg and foot anatomy will be encouraged to use it actively in a clinical setting. The ideal use of this book would perhaps be to prop it open next to an examination couch while the reader translates the page into practice with a colleague (or willing patient).

For the already inspired reader, the book should provide an ideal clinical counterpoint to the heavyweight anatomical titles, while for more hesitant reader it is sincerely hoped that the clinical flavour will help overcome any reticence they may have about developing a better understanding of basic leg and foot anatomy.

Anthony Redmond
Unit of Musculoskeletal Disease
University of Leeds, UK

Chapter 1

Palpation: principles and practice

Contents

Definitions and concepts	2
Palpation: definitions	2
General characteristics of palpation	2
Touch	2
General characteristics	2
The physiology of touch	3
The social significance of touch	4
Touch and clinical practice	5
Effects of palpation on the patient	6
Patient and person	6
The consultation process	7
Techniques of palpation	8
Improving the art of palpation	9
Care of the hands	10
Palpation of different tissues	10
Summary	12

DEFINITIONS AND CONCEPTS

Palpation: definitions

The Oxford Dictionary of English defines the verb 'to palpate' as: 'to examine (a part of the body) by touch, especially for medical purposes'. Its derivative noun is 'palpation' (from the Latin verb *palpare*: to 'feel or touch gently'.) According to *The Chambers Dictionary*, the term 'palp' means 'to feel, examine or explore by touch'; *palpare* is defined as 'to touch softly, stroke, caress or flatter'. *Churchill's Medical Dictionary* defines palpation as 'to stroke, caress; to explore or examine by touching and probing with the hands and fingers'.

Whilst 'stroking', 'caressing' or (tactile) 'flattering' represent practices (through 'gentle touch') that are essentially designed to give physiological and psychological 'healing' to the recipient, palpation, for the purposes of this text, is primarily a purposeful activity requiring considerable skill. It is associated with methodical exploration and detailed manual examination, the aim of which is to acquire objective information that will eventually lead to a reasoned medical diagnosis upon which a subsequent treatment regimen can be based. *Gould's Medical Dictionary* makes the direct link between the activity of palpation and diagnosis by gentle touch which involves the detection of the 'characteristics and condition of local tissues of the underlying organs or tumors'.

In *The Oxford Dictionary of English*, 'to examine' is defined as 'to test; to inquire into; to question; to look closely at or into; to inspect'. According to *The Chambers Dictionary*, 'to examine' is to 'inspect (someone or something) thoroughly in order to determine the nature of a condition'. The activity involves critical, reflective thinking: the systematic weighing up of evidence in an attempt to arrive at a balanced conclusion.

General characteristics of palpation

Palpation is a highly complex and sophisticated manual skill. Citing Frymann, Chaitow (2003) draws attention to the potential which palpation offers members of the healing professions:

> The human hand is equipped with instruments to perceive changes in texture, surface texture, surface humidity, to penetrate and detect successively deeper tissue textures, turgescence, elasticity and irritability. The human hand, furthermore, is designed to detect minute motion, motion which can only be detected by the most sensitive electronic pick-up devices available. This carries the art of palpation beyond the various modalities of touch into the realm of

proprioception, of changes in position and tension within our own muscular system.

(Chaitow 2003)

As Frymann emphasizes, the hand is particularly well equipped to play the key role in this activity. With reference to palpation of the human body, Chaitow reminds us that different parts of the hand possess the ability to discriminate between variations in tissue features: '... relative tension, texture, degree of moisture, temperature and so on.' He then makes the important point that 'This highlights the fact that an individual's overall palpatory sensitivity depends on a combination of different perceptive (and proprioceptive) qualities and abilities' (Chaitow 2003).

TOUCH

General characteristics

Palpation involves the use of one of the primary senses, that of touch, in order to investigate and obtain information or to supplement that already gained by other means, such as by visual and auditory input. As Poon (1995) points out:

> The act of touching and the feeling of being touched are very powerful experiences ... (and touch) is the earliest and most primitive form of communication.

(Poon 1995)

Montague (1978) reminds us that:

> Touch is the first of the senses to develop in the embryo and it plays a very important role in the birth process itself and in the early life of the individual.

(Montague 1978)

Not only is it the earliest system to become functional in the human being but touch is also thought to be the last of the senses to be lost immediately prior to death.

Touch plays a very significant part in our everyday experience:

> When the other senses are not wholly effective, we return to the sense of touch to rediscover reality. Clothing is felt to determine its quality, fruit is squeezed to determine its ripeness and paint is touched to test for dryness.

(Mason 1985)

Experience suggests, however, that there are instances when touch is often subjugated in favour of reliance upon other sensory modalities. Only when an awareness of an alteration in incoming stimuli occurs do we become conscious of the sense of touch. An example of this phenomenon might be when picking up a garment, we recognize its unfamiliarity through its texture or 'feel'; another example might be an awareness of the material of trousers touching the legs immediately after a long period of wearing shorts.

Touch may be divided into two distinct categories: instrumental and expressive. Touch is described as instrumental when it is associated with a deliberate action: locating an anatomical structure for the purposes of examination during a clinical assessment, for example. Touch is identified as expressive when it is associated with spontaneous, affective actions: touching a distressed person's arm in order to convey sympathy and offer comfort (MacWhannell 1992, Poon 1995).

Touch can be experienced as safe or unsafe; physically comfortable or uncomfortable. It can be used to establish rapport: hand-shaking as a formal greeting at the beginning of a clinical interview or as a means of ending a treatment session. Communication by touch is specifically permitted within particular interpersonal relationships (see later). In certain contexts, however, permission to touch may be required, for example, at the commencement, and during the various stages of a clinical examination and treatment session. Touch is associated with psychological reactions: it is difficult to touch or be touched by those who elicit negative responses. The anticipation of touching or being touched can increase stress levels and these reactions may be influenced by personality, cultural and social factors: some female patients may deliberately avoid consulting a male therapist; some patients may be reluctant to remove clothing. It is important to remember that professional personnel are placed in an extremely powerful and privileged position in relation to others: they are given a license to touch and this power and privilege should never be abused.

The physiology of touch

All areas of the skin supplied with appropriate receptors are normally able to perceive a variety of sensations (pain, degrees of pressure, temperature changes, etc.) to a greater or lesser degree. Some areas, however, are more sensitive to stimuli than others because:

> The degree of tactile sensitivity in any area is in direct proportion to the number of sensory units present and active in that area, as well as to the degree of overlap of their receptive fields, which vary in size. Small receptive fields with many sensory units therefore have the highest degree of discriminatory sensitivity.
>
> (Chaitow 2003)

Sensitivity to spatial discrimination is poor in the lumbar region, the legs and the back of the hands. In the back of the hands, for example, two points can only be perceived separately if they are more than 50–100 mm apart. The lips, tongue and fingertips, however, rate high (1–3 mm). Thus individuals with normal sensation in the fingertips should be able to distinguish between two points even when they are less than 6 mm apart. This is referred to as the 'Two Point Discrimination Test' (see Chaitow 2003, Evans 2000, Magee 1997). The significance of this is that only relatively large objects can be recognized by the receptors in the lumbar region whereas fine point discrimination can be achieved when employing the fingertips.

Chaitow makes the further point that:

> Not only is there a difference of perception relating to spatial accuracy, but also one relating to intensity. An indentation of 6 micrometers is capable of being registered on the finger pads, while 24 micrometers is needed before the sensors in the palm of the hand reach their threshold and perceive the stimulus.
>
> (Chaitow 2003)

Additionally, Evans (2000) contends that:

> Under normal conditions, touch is an exploratory sense rather than purely receptive, and it is becoming increasingly evident that tactile acuity is enhanced in active exploration when compared with passive reception.
>
> (Evans 2000)

Citing Meyers, Etherington and Ashcroft (1958) Evans suggests that:

> An early indication of the phenomenon may be seen in an examination of the parameters of perception required to read Braille. The dots are separated by 2.3 mm, which is close to the threshold value for two-point discrimination at the pad of the index finger. Reduction of the inter-dot space to 1.9 mm only moderately reduces the legibility of the Braille text.
>
> (Evans 2000)

While sighted Braille transcribers, relying solely on visual input, have been known to become proficient at reading Braille by the end of only three weeks, experience confirms that individuals attempting to conquer the system by touch are estimated to take an average of 1½–2 years to reach a speed suitable for serious study, even with regular practice. This is not due to lack of knowledge of the system; rather it is because the palpation and recognition of the signs using tactile input requires a considerable amount of dedicated time and practice in which to develop. As with all skills, the speed and quality of reading depends upon the frequency and amount of use. The ability to palpate with any finger or fingers can usually be developed, the use of the index finger being the most popular. Reading speed is further enhanced by using the fingers of both hands. In some cases, this skill never develops if the individual has not learnt to employ touch from an early age. In rare instances, people who have been unable to use their fingers have developed the same ability to read Braille by using their toes or even their lips! (see above). This means that, regardless of the method by which this skill is acquired, the ability to increase the information received through sensory input can be improved, given time and serious dedication to regular practice. This can be of great benefit to the clinical practitioner who wishes to 'read' information that lies deep to the skin. The controlled use of pressure and movement, coupled with feedback and experience, unlocks a vast quantity of information that is often unavailable to the eye.

Obtaining information through touch is a skill, the practical significance of which is often not fully appreciated or valued until it is needed, perhaps to compensate for the impairment or loss of one of the other senses: sight or hearing, for example. Because of this, considerable practice is often required before the skill of palpation becomes developed to the point where it is of practical use to the individual concerned (see above). Initially, new techniques have to be devised and then undertaken slowly and carefully, with regular practice and evaluation, often involving feedback from other observers with consequent modification of behaviour. Efforts to recognize and accurately interpret tactile sensory input demand high levels of concentration which necessarily cause anxiety and additional stress to an individual who is unaccustomed to placing such reliance on this variety of incoming stimuli. These reactions are likely to be experienced by the novice clinical practitioner as well as by the recently disabled person and should be regarded as normal responses to the process of acquiring a new range of sophisticated psychomotor skills and personal strategies (Owen Hutchinson, Atkinson and Orpwood 1998).

In other non-medical contexts, touch-related skills are used to acquire general information about the environment such as establishing the temperature of water. A thermometer could be employed for this purpose, but it is often easier (and quicker) to test water temperature by utilizing the input from the sensory endings in the skin. While the results of this method of temperature testing are likely to be far less accurate than if a thermometer were to be used, they provide a range of potentially significant information upon which subsequent action could be based. The water temperature, for example, might be experienced as burning, scorching, boiling, extremely hot, very hot, fairly hot, hot, quite hot, very warm, blood heat, warm, fairly warm, slightly warm, cool, cold, quite cold, very cold, bitterly cold, freezing and icy cold. A temperature of 42°C read from a thermometer has little practical meaning as to whether something is too hot or too cold to touch.

The social significance of touch

The concept of the novice engaged in learning to interpret incoming stimuli received through touch extends, of course, into the realm of social interaction. As suggested above, touch can represent a powerful means of expressive communication (Nathan 1999). The way in which this communication is interpreted will be contingent upon such variables as personality, upbringing, culture and social situation and, in these contexts, it seems unhelpful to separate touch into mechanical and psychosocial categories. Referring to a medical intervention, Nathan contends that:

> Touching a person's body in a non therapeutic context is not normally considered an act of merely mechanical significance. Nor is it a procedure of a technique – rather it is an act of self-expression, or occasionally self-assertion, or preservation.
>
> (Nathan 1999)

The degree to which people will engage in touching will be dictated by the nature of the interpersonal relationship in which they are involved at the time. Nathan continues:

> In the main, frequent touching is reserved for parent–child relationships, lovers and close friends. In these contexts it both signifies emotional intimacy and is emotionally significant.
>
> (Nathan 1999)

Touch can be employed to communicate a variety of emotions. For example, affection may be conveyed by a gentle squeeze of the hand whereas a loose handshake may imply indifference or even dislike. Touching and being touched can be extremely therapeutic. Montague summarizes the observations of many researchers who conclude that:

> Cutaneous stimulation in the various forms in which the newborn and young receive it is of prime importance for their healthy physical and behavioural development ... It appears probable that for human beings, tactile stimulation is of fundamental significance for development of healthy, emotional and affectional relationships.
>
> (Montague 1978)

Montague quotes examples of cases that were studied by Lorna Marshall, a researcher who spent much time between 1950 and 1961 living among the Bushmen of the Kalahari Desert in Botswana, South West Africa. He observed that, within this society, the development of the newborn, infant, adolescent and adult appeared to be influenced by the way in which the child was handled in early life. Montague also refers to accounts by Margaret Mead, who studied the Arapesh and Mundugumor societies in New Guinea during the 1930s and documented the characteristics of their respective social practices. In the former tribe, the child was in contact with the mother for most of the day. The adults of this tribe were observed to be kind, happy and peace-loving people. In the latter tribe, the child had little human contact, being kept in a rough plaited basket which was usually suspended from the mother's forehead. The adults of this tribe were observed to become unattractive, aggressive and cannibalistic.

The tendency to avoid close physical contact can be demonstrated in adults from certain cultures and within some social backgrounds of particular nationalities. Montague comments that 'There exists not only cultural and national differences in tactile behaviour but also class differences.' He cites the English upper class as a an example of a social group that is characterized by non-tactile social behaviour when compared with social groups of other nationalities: French and Italian people display more demonstrative behaviour when greeting one another and are observed to engage in more physical interpersonal contact.

When considering the practice of palpation skills, the significance of Montague's observations cannot be underestimated. Not only is it crucial for us to recognize the relevance of culture, nationality and social class on the degree to which people communicate by touch, but also the impact of living in a multicultural society in which we are likely to encounter unfamiliar and potentially disconcerting practices. Additionally the effect of globalization on our patterns of non-verbal communication has been considerable.

In contrast to the somewhat reserved behaviour of English people in the 19th and early 20th centuries, we now regularly witness overt instances of emotion (love and friendship, happiness and sadness) through physical contact. Behaviour such as mutual embracing, hand-holding and kissing is frequently to be observed in public places. Sports-people will leap in the air and hug each other following a winning achievement such as the scoring of a goal in football; equally, it is not uncommon for athletes to display tears of misery and frustration and to engage in mutually sympathetic embraces after a failure to attain high standards of performance.

Touch and clinical practice

Palpation, then, would seem to be a practice which involves a combination of many other skilled activities: the appropriate use of touch, the application of methodical investigatory techniques, accurate interpretation of sensory feedback (based upon sound general knowledge), the ability to draw on previous experience, to reflect, critically, upon findings and arrive at a reasoned conclusion.

> Palpation is the art of feeling tissues with your hands in such a manner that changes in tension and position within these tissues can be readily noticed, diagnosed and treated.
>
> (Mitchell, Moran and Pruzzo (1979)
> cited in Chaitow 2003)

A skill is attained and retained by its continual use, evaluation and modification of practice (Phillips 2004). The study and practice of manual contact techniques over a long period of time enables the practitioner to become highly skilled in the art of palpation. The development of this skill provides valuable supplementary information to that which can be obtained through observation and verbal questioning and is crucial to arriving at a meaningful clinical diagnosis. After many years experience of practising palpation skills, the moving, stretching and compression of tissues will be undertaken with precise control. This will enable the therapist to receive and interpret vital information from the patient and to apply and modify techniques as appropriate. Small changes in tension, temperature, dampness, movement and swelling will be identified by the sense of touch; these will then be noted and the appropriate course of action taken. Grieve states:

> Of the entire objective examination of the vertebral column, the palpation examination of accessible tissues is probably the most informative and therefore the most valuable.
>
> (Grieve 1986)

As has been noted above, however, learning to palpate is also associated with acquiring the skills to 'read', accurately, the patient's problem. Citing Ford (1989), Chaitow reminds us that:

> In days gone by, when a physician had to diagnose by touch a good practitioner did not feel a tumour at his fingertips but he projected his vibratory and pressure sensations into the patient. So we regularly project our sense of touch beyond our physical being and ... merely make the ordinarily unconscious process available to our conscious mind. In so doing, we cross the delicate boundary between self and other, to explore, to learn, and ultimately to help.
>
> (Chaitow 2003)

Personal experience confirms that patients can easily distinguish between a novice and an expert practitioner. During the initial examination, both the practitioner and the person being palpated progress through a learning process in which each is engaged in assessing the other by the giving and receiving of information. Relatively little significant information can be obtained if one of the participants in this relationship is reluctant to communicate. This learning process takes time and it is often the case that an accurate picture of the underlying issues does not appear until much later in the treatment session. The reason for this is partly due to the need for each participant to become comfortable with the other, so permitting mutual reduction in anxiety and the relaxation of tension. It is also due to the need for both parties to become familiar with the learning process itself, so that each can benefit from the knowledge gained as a result of their participation in this two-way event. The skill of palpation, therefore, should not be regarded merely as an arbitrary form of physical intervention; rather it must be respected as a highly skilled investigative process which elicits specialized information to both participants. In our experience, the skill of palpation is estimated to be only 10% innate: the other 90% is acquired through dedicated practice.

EFFECTS OF PALPATION ON THE PATIENT

Patient and person

It is far beyond the scope of this book to enter into the complexities of the mind–body debate, but its significance in relation to clinical diagnosis and management cannot be ignored. Traditionally, medical practice has been characterized by the biomedical model of health. This model is underpinned by the philosophical principles of dualism: the mind and body are regarded as separate and distinct entities that do not interact and, essentially, the practitioner is engaged in treating one or the other. The manual therapist would, in this context therefore, be regarded as being concerned only with the treatment of the patient's body. Indeed, it is not uncommon to hear therapists refer to a patient as 'a neck' or 'a back'. The body is considered to resemble a sophisticated machine; if part of that machine is malfunctioning, physical intervention is required in order to rectify the fault (Chaitow in Nathan 1999, Christensen, Jones and Edwards 2004, Owen Hutchinson 2004).

The 1990s, however, have witnessed significant changes in the approach towards illness and disability with the consequent development of the biopsycho-

social model of disability which 'is a way of conceptualizing the multifactorial and complex system that shapes a person's experiences of pain and disability' (Christensen, Jones and Edwards 2004.) Citing various sources, Christensen, Jones and Edwards explain the biopsychosocial theory:

> ... the degree of disability a person develops will be based upon the reactions of that person to the pain experienced far more than on the physical experience of the pain itself. The biopsychosocial model places a complaint of pain into a more holistic context, and views the pain as important not in isolation, but in relation to any disability the person with pain is experiencing as a result of that pain.
> (Christensen, Jones and Edwards 2004)

(See also Ramsden 1999, Stevenson, Grieves and Stein-Parbury 2004).

The last decade has also witnessed a growth in the popularity of complementary medicine, whose underlying holistic principles stand in direct contrast to those of orthodox medical practice. This trend would suggest that patients prefer to be treated as whole persons rather than as bodies requiring cures. When they seek consultation with a therapist, patients are asking for help with more than just a painful neck or back: they want far more than to be the passive recipient of skilfully performed physical techniques. Indeed, patients regard a satisfactory healing experience as one that acknowledges the inextricable links between mind and body and which therefore treats the whole person who is more than just the sum of a collection of constituent parts. Recognizing this, the therapist must adopt an empathic and sensitive approach to all input from the patient, both in terms of verbal and non-verbal communication. Social and cultural factors must also be taken into account.

The quality of all clinical interventions will improve dramatically if the person-centred approach to patient management is adopted. The therapist, however, should not underestimate the degree to which patients have learned the conventions associated with society in general and medicine in particular. During the session, patients will often choose to use language to conceal as well as to reveal emotional states: 'That movement does not hurt any more'; 'I feel much freer now'. It must always be remembered that the patient has this choice. It must also be borne in mind that some patients may not have recognized the link between physical and psychological states and may need to be encouraged to reflect upon their choice of language in order to gain insight into certain aspects of their emotional lives.

As has been suggested above, the act of touching and the feeling of being touched are very powerful experiences and the degree to which people engage in touching is largely contingent upon personality, cultural and social factors. Both patient and therapist may experience an increase in stress levels due to unfamiliarity within particular therapeutic contexts. The practitioner must demonstrate a respect for the patient as a person. Permission to touch should be obtained at the commencement, and during the various stages of a clinical intervention. Abuse of power and the privilege of being licensed to touch must be avoided.

The consultation process

For a variety of physical and psychosocial reasons, many patients remain reluctant to consult professional personnel on matters associated with their personal issues, especially those problems relating to their own bodies. Barriers may be erected by one or both participants in the therapist–patient relationship, although both must contribute to the dismantling of these barriers if effective communication and co-operation are to be achieved. Experience suggests that each patient usually presents with a combination of issues which are revealed by the identification of problems, the giving of information and the posing of a number of questions during the consultation process. Typically, no particular order of priority emerges except perhaps that associated with the overriding presence of pain. Some of the information provided by the patient may appear to be somewhat peripheral in relation to the practitioner's objective of establishing a clinical diagnosis, but it nevertheless represents a vital component of the overall clinical picture and must be thoroughly evaluated before it can be discounted.

The practitioner must be sympathetically receptive to all forms of information offered by the patient. Standards governing all areas of professional practice demand that the clinician must objectively evaluate all clinical evidence and attempt to produce a comprehensive analysis of the presenting situation. On some occasions, a prescribed plan will be used to facilitate the compilation and evaluation of data; at other times, the practitioner will be expected to tailor the procedure according to the patient's individual circumstances. The use of such strategies will enable the practitioner to arrive at a reasoned clinical diagnosis. Care must be taken, however, that any prescribed plan does not preclude the practitioner from obtaining relevant information from the patient; adherence to such standard proforma can sometimes adversely affect the practitioner's judgement and thus lead to an incorrect clinical assessment of the patient's current problem.

It is crucial that the practitioner should manage the initial investigation with great care and sensitivity as this process is likely to have a significant influence on both parties during the subsequent clinical examination. The practitioner should exercise the same degree of tact and diplomacy when conducting the subsequent physical examination, which should be undertaken with equal care, precision and gentleness. Physical or verbal clumsiness at this stage of the proceedings could lead to a complete breakdown of the interpersonal relationship between the therapist and patient, who may become reluctant to communicate vital information. The therapist employs palpation techniques during the first contact with the patient and it is vital that efficient methods of obtaining information are employed at this time. Experience suggests that most patients have an expectation that a clinical examination involving the use of palpation techniques will take place; indeed, they would consider it to be unprofessional practice if such a procedure were not undertaken. Inevitably, each person will exhibit different reactions to being touched and it is important that the practitioner should establish and evaluate the patient's unique reaction to such interventions at the earliest opportunity. An initial indication of the patient's reaction to physical contact can be obtained by the act of hand-shaking at the commencement of the session. Additionally, information gained by the act of assisting the patient to and from a chair can provide the practitioner with valuable feedback relating to the patient's degree of willingness or reluctance to accept help. Of course, such strategies represent only part of the range of techniques being employed during this initial session. The use of visual, auditory and olfactory input can also provide useful sources of relevant clinical information.

During the period of questioning, the practitioner is recommended to make sensitive and careful physical contact with the area of the patient's pain. When these techniques are performed successfully, this encourages both parties to focus attention on the patient's motivation in seeking the consultation. All movements should be tested carefully, palpation skills being employed simultaneously with continual observation of the ongoing situation, the therapist monitoring any reluctance on the part of the patient to perform movements due to tension, muscle spasm, joint anomalies and pain. Inadvertently eliciting symptoms of acute pain will inevitably destroy the patient's confidence, resulting in an unwillingness to offer potentially significant information.

In most cases, the patient will gradually gain confidence and learn to trust the practitioner. Much of the apprehension of meeting will have passed during the initial contact. When the time comes for the therapist to undertake an objective physical examination of the patient's movements, rapport should have been well established which overcomes that initial reluctance to seeking of medical advice.

Palpation continues throughout the examination and subsequent treatment. If it is carried out carefully and sympathetically, it reveals valuable information concerning the patient's physical and psychological condition. Indeed, palpation has the potential to 'unlock' psychological issues which had hitherto been deliberately ignored or unrecognized by the patient as having any relevance to the presenting physical problem. Many practitioners will have experience of patients who seek medical consultation for a relatively minor physical ailment which, during the examination or treatment, will be found to be masking much deeper and more complex issues. All practitioners should be sensitive to this possibility and should note any incongruous sentiments that the patient may express during the session. Experience suggests that it is the physical contact with the patient which appears to facilitate the unveiling of these underlying issues but the importance of recognizing this phenomenon is contingent upon the quality of the practitioner's professional training.

That the patient must have confidence in the practitioner cannot be over-emphasized. This will promote the offering of information through both verbal and non-verbal communication methods. Throughout the consultation, the practitioner should be receptive to the patient; as the session progresses, continual evaluation of the patient's verbal and non-verbal reactions to events should take place. Whether complex or simple, all treatment sessions should promote mutual trust and understanding. Experience indicates that the degree to which a patient contributes to the treatment session is directly proportional to the practitioner's input; this reciprocal relationship is, however, contingent on the practitioner's willingness to impart information and the patient's genuine interest in receiving it.

TECHNIQUES OF PALPATION

It is not enough merely to place the hands on the patient's body and hope to receive the information required. Positive steps must be taken to search for the data. As has been noted above, palpation is associated with the seeking of information and all techniques must be approached in a rational and logical manner. The practitioner can gain very little by contacting a surface with the hands and remaining stationary. Movement of the hands is required so that structures can pass under the fingers in a controlled manner so that any alterations in skin temperature, surface

tension, and bone structure can be evaluated and recorded. The practitioner's speed of movement can be adjusted to facilitate the full interpretation of information. The importance of regularly modifying the speed of movement can be demonstrated by the following example. If the fingers are run over Braille script too quickly, dots can be felt but no information is obtained; if the individual adapts the speed accordingly, however, what initially appeared to be an incomprehensible mass of dots now becomes an intelligible text.

Sometimes palpation techniques need to be performed slowly and at considerable depth; at other times they should be carried out quickly and at a superficial level. For example, palpation of the transverse processes of the spines of the lumbar region or the hook of the hamate needs careful application of deep pressure, combined with slow movement and sensitivity to the patient's reactions. Palpation of the spines of the thoracic vertebrae – particularly when counting downwards – is much easier if the fingertips are gently moved up and down three or four centimetres at a time, marking each spine with the finger of the other hand and holding it until the position of the next spine is confirmed. This type of palpation works in a similar way to a scanner using a beam to build up a clearer picture. The technique can be used to obtain a clearer picture of the rib cage, particularly from the posterior aspect.

In our experience, using one or even two complete palms and fingertips conveys more information regarding movement below the skin surface and about the patient's general reaction to physical contact than if the fingertips alone were used. The application of the fingertips alone, for example, would be used for palpating a pulse. Generally, if the structures below the surface are stationary, the hands will have to be used in a controlled movement, whereas if the structures are mobile, the hands should remain stationary. The finer the movement below the surface, the more delicate the palpation technique must be: this is clearly demonstrated when searching for a faint pulse.

If joints are being manipulated to examine the quality of movement and to assess limiting factors, the hands should be moved as little as possible so as to avoid any feedback from the palpator's own tissues which would obscure information from those of the patient. In fact, with this kind of palpation, a minimum of all other movements – with the exception of the joint being examined – is required. This involves adopting a stance which will avoid movement of the feet, applying a hold that will allow the full range of movement without change and also reducing all skin sliding by firm contact. Finally, the palpator must be absolutely sure that the patient's position is stable and that the movement being tested is localized to the joint being examined and is in the plane around the axis required. It is not uncommon, when testing the movements of the upper or lower limb, for a 'clicking' or crepitus to occur and neither the patient nor the examiner are able to locate its source. Conversely, if the examiner's thumb nails touch when pressure is being applied to the posterior aspect of the lateral mass of the atlas (C1), the patient may, erroneously, report a grinding sound located in the atlanto-occipital joint.

When examining the end-range of a joint, all variations must be known in advance so that movement, physiological and accessory, is tested accurately, noting the range available and the limiting factors. This is a highly skilled form of palpation, requiring a great deal of practice on normal joints in order to perfect the technique, considerable experience with abnormal joints to be able to recognize the variations and an expert knowledge of the various conditions to assess how much or how little testing should be undertaken. It is not suggested that this form of palpation should be employed by an expert only; on the contrary, the technique should be practised at the earliest opportunity and based on palpation of normal anatomy. Gradually, if care is taken and limits set, considerable skill can be gained.

Experience suggests that some palpators either under-employ the use of touch and try to compensate by observation, or they tend to palpate over-enthusiastically but fail to interpret the significance of what they feel. Some may also feel what they believe they are meant to feel. It is easy to be persuaded by an eager patient, by prior knowledge or by a more experienced observer that one can feel changes that are not actually present. An open and honest interpretation of what is beneath the fingertips is essential: remember Hans Andersen's story of the Emperor's new clothes!

IMPROVING THE ART OF PALPATION

Returning to the example of the Braille reader, improvement in palpation techniques can only be achieved with practice. As with all areas of knowledge, the motivation to learn is crucial. In relation to clinical practice, the learning of good palpation skills is contingent upon the need to know what lies beneath the surface of the body and the desire to find some means of offering help to patients. Practitioners frequently express the wish to be able to 'see what is happening beneath the surface'. These sentiments confirm the importance of developing appropriate palpation techniques which can then be employed as a means of providing assistance. Inextricably linked with this process is the development of manual dexterity and sensitivity.

It is worth noting that, when practising any technique that necessarily involves the use of the hands, the quality of the information that is received through the sense of touch can often be enhanced by reducing the input from the other senses. Closing the eyes and using the hands to recognize different textures, weights, surfaces, liquids, coins, etc. often reveals hitherto unrecognized characteristics of what are regarded as familiar objects. The palpator must endeavour to obtain as much information from the sense of touch as possible. In order to develop this skill, different objects can be placed in a bag and identified only by using the hands. As the skill improves, less familiar objects can be chosen so that they are less recognizable: their shape might be more unusual and/or they may be smaller. All of these objects should be handled sensitively by the palpator who should attempt to identify their distinctive features (such as blemishes). Progression of this exercise would be to require the palpation and identification of the same objects through the material of the bag. The material of the bag could be chosen so that the exercise becomes progressively more difficult: beginning with a relatively thin surface such as fine plastic and gradually changing to a thicker material. Practise should be undertaken regularly during the course of everyday activities, the practitioner always noting the technique which is most suitable for the identification of each object. One suggestion would be habitually to identify the loose change in a pocket or purse before removing the correct amount to make a purchase. Recognition of coins is a relatively easy task and it should be unnecessary to use vision in order to verify the amount tendered. Take care: this could prove to be an expensive way to learn the art of palpation if adequate practice is not undertaken! Another exercise might be to select clothing on a daily basis using tactile and not visual input. It is a salutary point that all visually impaired people necessarily employ these tactual skills every day.

The development of the sense of touch needs to be nurtured. It is recommended that each contact with an object should be treated as if no visual or auditory input is available whilst attempting to obtain the maximum amount of information. Those who have the privilege of handling patients professionally possess a constant source of practice in their study of structure and function and examination of normal and abnormal phenomena. Those professionals are even more fortunate if they specialize in the use of massage, movement, mobilization and manipulation techniques as part of clinical practice. Individuals who have undertaken formal study and practice of the art of massage are indeed already well versed in the appropriate knowledge and skills relating to palpation. Their contribution to the increased public recognition of palpation as a crucial element in the diagnosis and treatment of clinical conditions cannot be underestimated. Indeed it is gratifying to note the increased status of all the manual therapies during the past decade: people are deliberately selecting practitioners who possess skills that rely on touch for their efficacy. It should never be forgotten, however, that all such therapists are required to demonstrate a serious commitment to Continuing Professional Development (CPD): they are required to revise and update their anatomical and physiological knowledge on a regular basis in order to maintain the high standards of professional practice demanded by their respective professional organizations.

CARE OF THE HANDS

All skills in which complex manual techniques are employed in the performance of precise movements, necessarily rely on the regular care and maintenance of the hands: their mobility, sensitivity and dexterity. Prior to engaging in any form of manual contact, however, the practitioner should ensure that the temperature of the skin is warm; patients do not appreciate being touched by therapists whose hands are cold!

Cleanliness is essential and its positive contribution to the quality of tactile input cannot be underestimated. Traces of grease, cream, dirt, dust, etc. effectively create an additional intervening layer between the sensory receptor organs and nerve endings in the hand and the object or subject to be palpated. It is significant that most Braille readers will make every effort to keep their hands clean while reading Braille; many tend to avoid eating anything sticky in order to prevent their fingers from losing sensitivity. A routine of washing the hands in warm water using a mild soap and drying them thoroughly after washing should be adopted, The use of additional creams or ointments is not recommended unless this is absolutely necessary. A good, oil-based hand cream can be used at night in order to maintain a smooth, soft condition of the skin; some authorities also recommend the regular use of Vaseline and sugar. Whichever maintenance routine is adopted, the hands must always be washed thoroughly prior to attempting palpation techniques. In addition, the nails should be kept clean and short so that the risks of injury or infection are avoided. No wrist or hand jewellery should be worn. The quality of the palpation depends, to a great extent, upon the texture and suppleness of the hands. They should look and feel good, thus promoting the patient's confidence in the palpator. Poorly maintained hands which are dirty, stiff and with hard skin will be off-putting to patients: a reluctance to be touched will act as a barrier to the passage of information from the body of the patient to the receptors of the palpator.

The joints of the hands must be maintained in a supple condition with the musculature being firm and strong. Regular exercises should be practised in order to maintain joint mobility and increase muscle strength. Contact with all abrasive surfaces and detergents should be avoided as far as possible and gloves should be worn at all times when manual work is performed, particularly during activities such as washing-up, cleaning, gardening, car maintenance and building work. Many liquids, certain soaps and detergents, tend to remove the natural greases from the skin and the use of these should, therefore, be minimal. Any activity that is likely to lead to the production of blisters, finger calluses or general hard skin should also be minimized: examples might include such pastimes as rowing, playing a stringed musical instrument, rope-climbing and woodwork. Additionally, great care must be taken when using sharp instruments or engaging in any activity that is likely to cause trauma and/or skin infection. Lack of vigilance whilst performing any of these activities may prejudice the ability to perform high-quality palpation techniques.

PALPATION OF DIFFERENT TISSUES

Experience suggests that normal palpation when performed by the lay person – and even when undertaken by some professionals – is sometimes ineffective. It may enable the operator to differentiate between such tissues as bone, muscle or tendon etc. but often does little more. By contrast, the skilled student practitioner will be able to distinguish different parts of bones, contrasting shapes and texture of muscles, identify their connections to tendons and trace them to their attachments. Such students will also be able to count vertebrae, palpate lumbar transverse processes and other deep bony structures, locate certain ligaments, palpate elusive pulses and determine abnormalities such as different types of swelling, misalignment and rupture. The expert clinician must progress far beyond this concept in order to complete the picture that lies hidden within the body. Bony landmarks should be studied, linking them together and obtaining a clear mental image of the skeletal layout. This programme should include studying rib angles, transverse processes and spines of all vertebrae including their differing features. For example, the bifid spinous processes of the cervical region contrast with the pointed spines in the thoracic and the rectangular-shaped spines of T12 and in the lumbar region. Alignment of one bone to another is relatively easily examined in the upper and lower limbs whereas this is much more difficult to examine in the vertebral column. Defects in the contour of a bone can also be located and possible avulsions recognized.

Variations in muscle texture should be identifiable and note taken of differences occurring in normal muscle, enabling the examiner to recognize any abnormal variations. Some muscles, such as gluteus maximus and the middle fibres of deltoid, have a coarse structure due to the type of muscle fibres involved, whereas muscles such as the oblique abdominals and quadratus lumborum have a smoother texture. Fibrous tissue between the muscle fibres may give a stringy feel, while local areas of spasm are hard but regular in shape. The former tend to remain in the same position irrespective of what technique is performed on them; the latter will often disappear on applying either heat or massage. Both types of muscle spasm can be found in the rhomboid muscles between the scapula and spinous processes of the vertebral column.

Careful palpation will reveal where each muscle joins its tendon and where and how the tendon is attached. Palpation can also determine how tightly the muscle is bound down by fascia and whether the tendon is maintained in its position by a retinaculum. The extent of the retinacula can be examined and a study made of those structures which pass under or over them.

Swellings in muscle are often caused by bruising (contusion) and bleeding (haematoma) between the muscle fibres. These are normally contained within a localized area and become hard and painful, often warm to the touch and sometimes produce redness over the area. There is nearly always a history of trauma to the region. Care should be taken, however, when palpating any area of swelling as this symptom could be caused by other more serious conditions. It is important to be sensitive to local changes in temperature, noting whether these are higher or lower than expected. The condition of the underlying structures must be recorded and a knowledge of the possible causes of such variations will contribute to the establishment of a clinical diagnosis and subsequent treatment of the condition.

When palpating joints, other considerations must be taken into account. The precise location of the joint line is essential, the quality of this technique being based on the accurate identification of bony landmarks and measurements, taking into account the general size and shape of other bones and the patient's posture

at the time. A detailed knowledge of the structure and extent of the adjacent joint surfaces, as well as where ligaments may obscure the joint space, is essential. The presentation of tissue-filled joint spaces under differing circumstances – for example, whether fluid is contained within the joint capsule or within a bursa – together with a detailed knowledge of the surrounding tendons is also a necessary pre-requisite when examining joints. As Chaitow points out:

> There are many important features to note during the examination of joints: the range and smoothness of movement, whether the axis varies according to the position of the joint and to what degree movement may be limited. Employing great care and skill, movement of joints can be examined indirectly through the bones of either side of that joint. The movement between the joint surfaces may be experienced as smooth or grinding; the restriction felt at the end of a joint's range of motion may be described as having a certain feel and this is called (the) 'end-feel'.
>
> (Chaitow 2003)

In his discussion of barriers to joint movement Chaitow continues:

> If there is, for any reason, a restriction in the range of motion then a pathological barrier would be apparent on active or passive movement in that direction. If the reason for the restriction involved interosseous changes (arthritis, for example) the end-feel would be sudden or hard. However, if the restriction involved soft tissue dysfunction the end-feel would have a softer nature.
>
> (Chaitow 2003)

Most joints possess additional movements which are of small range and not under voluntary control: these are essential for the efficient functioning of the joint. These are known as 'accessory' movements.

> Accessory or joint play movements are those movements of a joint that cannot be performed actively by the individual. Such accessory movements include the roll, spin and slide which accompany a joint's physiological movements.
>
> (Hengeveld and Banks 2005)

A simple example of this type of movement would be found in the axle of a bicycle wheel. On each side, the axle is surrounded by a ring of ball-bearings maintained in position by a cone which screws on to the axle. When the cones are loose, they allow the wheel to be moved slightly from side to side; when the cones are tight, there is no side-to-side or accessory movement. When there is side-to-side movement, the wheel is free to turn; as the cones are tightened, the ball-bearings become 'close packed' and more difficult to turn so finally locking the wheel. The side-to-side (or accessory) movement is thus essential for the free turning of the wheel, since its elimination results in no movement.

Accessory movements are most demonstrable in human joints within a certain range of the joint movement: when the ligaments allow joint surfaces to be parted or when the surfaces are not congruent. This is termed the 'loose packed' position. When the ligaments of a joint become taut and its surfaces are congruent, no further movement is possible, either physiological or accessory. The joint is now said to be in a 'close packed' position (Standing 2004). If the accessory movements of a joint are lost, the joint becomes extremely difficult to move, similar to the cones of the bicycle wheel being tightened (see above). If, however, accessory movement is restored, as in loosening the cones in the bicycle wheel, normal movement is also restored. The restoration of accessory movements is an important principle underlying the practice of mobilization and manipulation techniques to restore normal movement in joints. With care and expertise, by using a combination of accessory and *normal* movements, joint function can be assessed and the treatment varied accordingly. The use of 'quadrant' techniques (combined movements at the end of range) is a good example of this testing. (For further information on the application of these types of examination and techniques, see Grieve 1986, Hengeveld and Banks 2005.)

Chaitow's definition of 'joint play' is also useful:

> Joint play refers to the particular movements between bones associated with either separation of the surfaces (as in traction) or parallel movement of joint surfaces (also known as translation or translatoric gliding).
>
> (Chaitow 2003)

This information is important in establishing the joints' condition.

Swelling around a joint deforms its shape and contour, the extent of the deformity being dependent upon the degree of swelling involved. The bony features can usually be identified between the areas of swelling. In some instances, the swelling is so profuse that it is difficult to locate bony landmarks; on other occasions, the amount of fluid is so small that precise techniques have to be employed to palpate the swelling which is interfering with normal joint function. Most joint swelling is contained within the capsule, causing a build-up of pressure which results in increasing pain. The swelling may have to be

removed surgically, although this is usually deferred until absolutely necessary because of the risk of infection into the joint. Blood can also escape into a joint space (haemarthrosis), resulting in a similar appearance, but this is usually accompanied by some discoloration and an increased local temperature. Any swelling can lead to severe damage to the mechanics of the joint; this damage may vary according to the type of fluid involved.

Careful palpation of the swelling can produce more information than at first thought. The swelling may appear soft and movable with the application of pressure; this often gives a fluid feel as it passes from one part of the joint cavity to another. Alternatively it may appear thick and pliable although difficult to move unless sustained pressure is applied. Swelling may appear to be a solid mass, pitting under pressure from the fingers but taking a considerable time before signs of movement are evident.

SUMMARY

Palpation is a detailed examination using the hands as tools to enable the palpator to elicit information about structures beneath the skin and fascia. It is, in our opinion, still under-used and under-valued, mainly because of lack of practise and appreciation of its intrinsic value. In addition, its teaching and practice are time-consuming, requiring expert instruction from experienced practitioners, genuine interest, patience and commitment from students. While its techniques can be practised and developed, however, expertise takes time and dedication to acquire.

Palpation is more than just a desire to 'see' through the skin and interpret the underlying anatomy. It can be developed in such a way that information can be imparted to the patient through the practitioner's hands. It is not difficult to appreciate the ways in which the expert palpator can employ the art of instrumental and expressive touching in combination to obtain clinical diagnosis and establish sympathetic communication. Indeed, the philosophy that underpins the practice of many therapists emphasizes the intrinsic therapeutic qualities of touch per se. (See for example Dennis, Jones and Holey 1995, Everett 1997, Nathan 1999, Charman 2000). Healers who practise the 'laying on of hands' and Therapeutic Touch also share this belief. (See Krieger 1986, 1993, 1997, 2002, Macrae 1987, Sayre-Adams and Wright 2001.) The increasing popularity of complementary therapies amongst the general public further confirms the general tendency to place considerable value in an holistic approach to patient care. Rather than relying solely on orthodox medical practice, patients and therapists alike are now recognizing the importance of healing in the management of chronic physical and psychological problems (Nathan 1999, Charman 2000).

Palpation must be learned, practised and developed before it can be applied professionally. The study of anatomy, physiology and the human sciences, together with the additional information obtained through the appropriate use of touch are excellent ways of learning the art of palpation. Anatomy will become clearer and more understandable as the hands become more sensitive to what lies below the skin, leading to an enhancement of knowledge and improvement in assessment: an asset in therapeutic application. Finally, and perhaps most importantly, the skilled palpator should be aware of the patient's reaction to movement. By observing the patient's face, listening to the patient's comments and being sensitive to all reactions in muscle and joint movement, a total picture of the patient's condition becomes available. With care and sensitivity, a great deal of information can easily be obtained.

The following chapters contain a detailed study of the surface markings of the structures of the lower limb, including a guide to the palpation of particular areas. It must be remembered, however, that the development of effective palpation skills for the purposes of clinical intervention requires more than the acquisition of sound theoretical knowledge upon which to base practice. As Chaitow emphasizes, expertise in palpation techniques is achieved '... by application (and repetition) of hundreds of carefully designed exercises that are capable of refining palpation skills to an astonishing degree of sensitivity' (Chaitow 2003).

Citing Frymann (1963) he adds:

> ... palpation cannot be learned by reading or listening; it can only be learned by palpation. This learning process is not just about hard dedicated labour; it should be fun and it should be exciting. The thrills to be experienced when taking this journey of exploration of the tissues of the human body is hopefully contagious ...
>   (Chaitow 2003)

We hope that readers will take inspiration from this and other related texts and strive to attain expertise in palpation skills in the interests of improving the quality of their clinical practice.

Chapter 2
Bones

Contents

The lumbar spine and pelvis	16
The thoracic outlet	16
The pelvic girdle	17
The lumbar vertebrae	18
The sacrum	18
The coccyx	19
The hip region	20
The knee region	24
Anterior aspect	25
Medial aspect	26
Lateral aspect	28
Posterior aspect	30
The ankle region	32
The lower end of the tibia	32
The lower end of the fibula	32
The talus	32
The calcaneus	33
The calcaneus	34
The foot	36
Dorsal aspect	36
Plantar aspect	38
Self-assessment questions	40

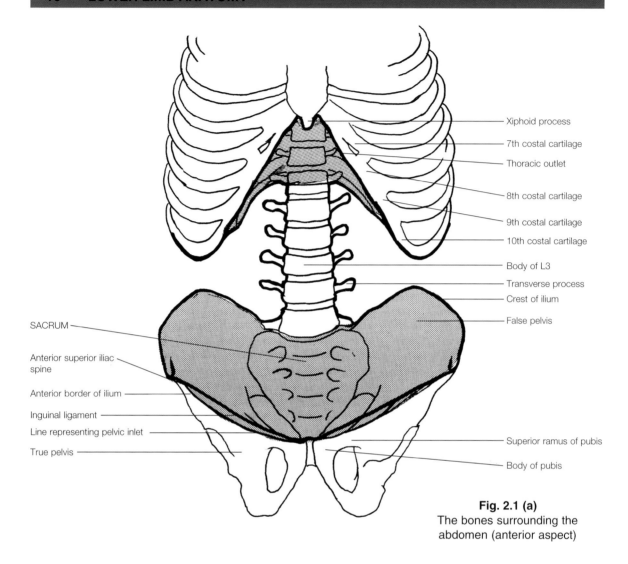

Xiphoid process

7th costal cartilage

Thoracic outlet

8th costal cartilage

9th costal cartilage

10th costal cartilage

Body of L3

Transverse process

Crest of ilium

False pelvis

SACRUM

Anterior superior iliac spine

Anterior border of ilium

Inguinal ligament

Line representing pelvic inlet

True pelvis

Superior ramus of pubis

Body of pubis

Fig. 2.1 (a)
The bones surrounding the abdomen (anterior aspect)

THE LUMBAR SPINE AND PELVIS

The abdomen consists mainly of soft tissue contained within predominantly muscular walls. Its only bony features are the boundaries of the **thoracic outlet** above consisting of the **xiphoid process** at its centre in the front, the lower border of the **seventh, eighth, ninth** and **tenth costal cartilages**, the tip of the eleventh rib and the inferior border of the twelfth rib. Posteriorly, the body of the twelfth thoracic vertebra completes the ring. Below, the pelvic inlet comprises the pubis anteriorly, its **superior rami** on either side, the **anterior border** and the **crest** of the **ilium** and posteriorly the **base of the sacrum**. The vertebral column forms its posterior boundary. It is, however, important to mark out these boundaries, as they provide useful landmarks for some of the organs it contains.

The thoracic outlet [Fig. 2.1a]

Palpation

Find the xiphoid process, which is the most inferior portion of the sternum. Trace along the costal margin beyond the costal angle (the ninth costal cartilage) to its lowest extremity, which is normally the **tenth rib**. Continuing posteriorly, the eleventh rib becomes evident, with its tip just anterior to the mid-axillary line, with the tip of the twelfth rib slightly lower and just posterior. The tip of the twelfth rib normally lies on the same level as the spine of the first lumbar vertebra.

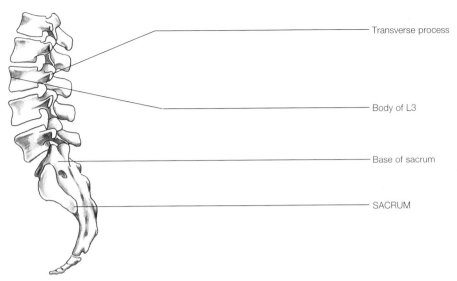

Transverse process

Body of L3

Base of sacrum

SACRUM

Fig. 2.1 (b)
The bones surrounding the abdomen (lateral aspect, viewed from left)

The pelvic girdle

Palpation

Identify the **anterior superior iliac spine** at the anterior extremity of the iliac crest. Trace the lateral lip of the iliac crest posteriorly, beyond the iliac tubercle to the posterior superior iliac spine and sacrum. Now, run the pads of your fingers down the central part of the abdominal wall to about 5 cm above the genitalia. The pubic tubercles become evident on either side, with each pubic crest running medially to a central space which marks the pubic symphysis. The bony ring is completed by the superior ramus of the pubis, which is difficult to palpate, and anterior border of the ilium, easily identifiable in its upper section. The **inguinal ligament** stretches above this region from the pubic tubercle to the anterior superior iliac spine.

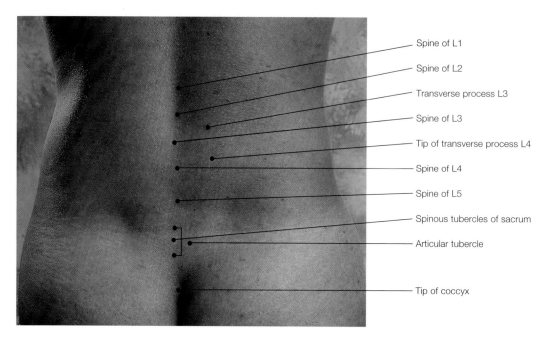

Spine of L1

Spine of L2

Transverse process L3

Spine of L3

Tip of transverse process L4

Spine of L4

Spine of L5

Spinous tubercles of sacrum

Articular tubercle

Tip of coccyx

Fig. 2.1 (c)
The lumbar vertebrae and sacrum (posterior aspect)

The lumbar vertebrae

There are five lumbar vertebrae, with L1 being the smallest and L5 the largest. As in all other vertebrae, their bodies are anterior and their spines are posterior. Laterally, they present **transverse processes**, the fifth being much larger than the rest. Their upper articular processes face inwards and their lower facets face outwards, those of the fifth facing more anteriorly. There is a large neural canal in the lumbar region which is more triangular in shape.

Palpation

Lumbar vertebrae. Posteriorly the spines of the lumbar vertebrae project backwards and are individually identifiable. With the subject lying prone, place a firm pillow under the abdomen which flattens the lumbar lordosis. This makes the spines of the lumbar vertebrae become more pronounced, appearing as a line of flattened edges forming a crest down the centre of the lumbar region (Fig. 2.1c,d). The spines are continuous with those of the sacrum below and the thoracic vertebrae above.

Immediately above the central part of the sacrum is a hollow, due to the spine of the fifth vertebra being shorter and the body being situated slightly more anterior than the rest. The small gaps between the spines tend to disappear when the vertebral column is flexed, owing to the tension of the supraspinous ligament.

If deep pressure is applied approximately 5 cm lateral to the vertebral spines, beyond the bulk of the erector spinae muscles, the tips of the transverse processes, particularly of the first lumbar vertebra, can be palpated. These are quite thin compared with those of the thorax and may be tender to palpate.

The sacrum

The **sacrum** is composed of five fused vertebrae, with S1 being the largest and S5 being the smallest. The sacrum is triangular in shape, with its base uppermost. Evidence of the separate vertebral bodies is still clear on the anterior surface. A line of spinous tubercles can be seen running vertically down the centre of its posterior surface and it is marked on either side by **articular tubercles**. Laterally the sacrum presents large lateral masses beyond its neural foramina. The sacrum is tilted forwards above, with its lower section projecting backwards.

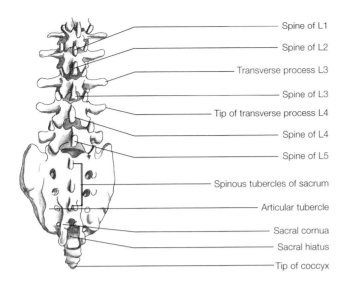

Spine of L1
Spine of L2
Transverse process L3
Spine of L3
Tip of transverse process L4
Spine of L4
Spine of L5
Spinous tubercles of sacrum
Articular tubercle
Sacral cornua
Sacral hiatus
Tip of coccyx

Fig. 2.1 (d)
The lumbar vertebrae and sacrum (posterior aspect)

Palpation

The sacrum. The posterior surface of the sacrum can be identified between the posterior borders of the two ilia. Its lower section projects backwards and is easy to palpate, while its upper section (the base) lies more anterior and is more difficult to examine. It has a central, vertical series of spinous tubercles, in line with the lumbar spines and the coccyx, accompanied on either side by a row of articular tubercles which are all palpable (Fig. 2.1c,d).

The coccyx

The coccyx comprises three or four rudimentary vertebrae normally fused into one bone, with the upper being the largest and the lowest being a very small tubercle of bone. Normally it is tilted, with its inferior tip pointing downwards and forwards.

Palpation

The coccyx. As this bone varies considerably in size and shape it may prove a little difficult to palpate. Several alternative methods can be employed:

1. Trace the spinous processes which run down the centre of the posterior surface of the sacrum to approximately 2.5 cm below the level of the posterior inferior iliac spines (see pages 22 and 23). Here, the pointed lower end of the coccyx can be palpated.
2. Gently run your fingers up the cleft between the two gluteus maximus muscles until the hard bony tip of the coccyx is found.
3. Draw an equilateral triangle with its base on the two posterior inferior iliac spines of the ilium with its apex downwards. This point should be on the tip of the coccyx.

In many subjects the coccyx is angled forwards and the finger must be pressed deep into the cleft to identify the shape. Care must be taken as pressure on the bone can cause pain, particularly if the joints between it and the sacrum have been damaged at any time.

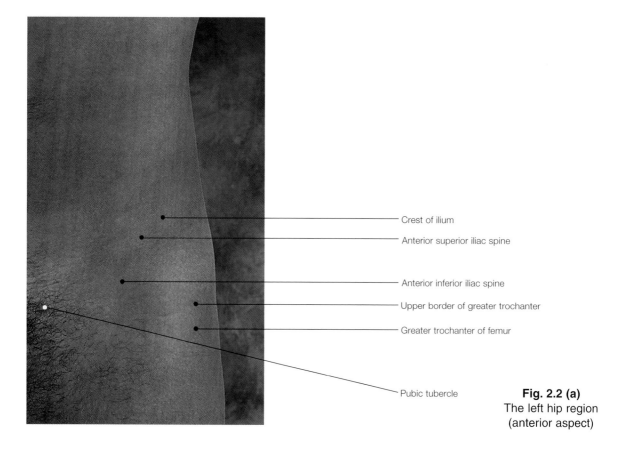

Crest of ilium

Anterior superior iliac spine

Anterior inferior iliac spine

Upper border of greater trochanter

Greater trochanter of femur

Pubic tubercle

Fig. 2.2 (a)
The left hip region
(anterior aspect)

THE HIP REGION

The two hip bones on either side and the sacrum, posteriorly, form the pelvic girdle. In its lower section it forms a complete ring (the true pelvis) with the two pubic bones joined at the pubic symphysis, whereas in its upper part (the false pelvis) the two blades of the **ilium** leave a large space anteriorly.

The hip or innominate bone (os innominatum (L) = bone without a name), comprises the ilium, the **ischium** and the **pubis**. They are united at the acetabulum, a deep rounded hollow situated on the lateral side of the bone on the constricted area between two blades. That above and posterior is the ilium and that below and anterior is the pubis and ischium. The ilium has an inner and outer surface with a broad crest above a narrow border at the front and back and the upper part of the sciatic notch inferiorly just posterior to its junction with the ischium. The lower blade presents a large **foramen**, medial to which is the flattened bone of the body of the pubis with a superior ramus above and an inferior ramus passing downwards and laterally. The ischium is situated below the acetabulum and forms the lateral part of the **obturator foramen** with its

ramus passing from below upwards to join the inferior ramus of the pubis.

The upper end of the femur comprises the **head, neck, greater and lesser trochanter**. The head lies medially and articulates in the acetabulum, the greater trochanter lies at the lateral end of the neck and the lesser trochanter projects medially and backwards from just below the junction of the neck with the shaft.

Palpation

Owing to the size and thickness of muscle and fascia, this region is much more difficult to investigate than the shoulder. It is often covered by a layer of fat, particularly in women, and this also adds to the difficulty in observation and palpation.

Face the subject, who is standing, and place both hands around the waist. On sliding the hands downwards a bony ridge, the **iliac** [ilium (L) = the flank] **crest,** is encountered on either side. Each can be traced forwards to end in a well-defined projection, the **anterior superior iliac spines** (ASIS) (Fig. 2.2). In lean

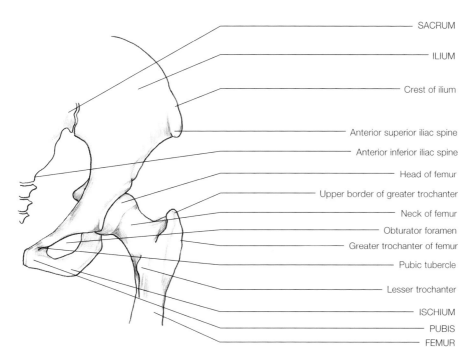

- SACRUM
- ILIUM
- Crest of ilium
- Anterior superior iliac spine
- Anterior inferior iliac spine
- Head of femur
- Upper border of greater trochanter
- Neck of femur
- Obturator foramen
- Greater trochanter of femur
- Pubic tubercle
- Lesser trochanter
- ISCHIUM
- PUBIS
- FEMUR

Fig. 2.2 (b)
Bones of the left hip region
(anterior aspect)

subjects the iliac crest is easily palpated from the ASIS to the posterior superior iliac spine (PSIS). In its anterior two-thirds it is convex laterally, broad and rounded, with inner and outer lips. Five to seven centimetres posterior to the ASIS, on its lateral lip, the tubercle of the crest is easily palpable, giving attachment to the upper end of the iliotibial tract. In its posterior third the iliac crest is concave laterally, less well defined and a little sharper on its superior border. The ASISs are set approximately 30 cm apart, a little more in the female, the abdomen usually protruding forwards between the two. From the ASIS, the sharp concave anterior border of the ilium can be traced downwards to another, less well-defined anterior projection, the **anterior inferior iliac spine** (AIIS), which lies approximately 2 cm above the rim of the acetablum (Fig. 2.2).

Now place the palm of your hand on the lower abdomen, moving it gently downwards; another ridge of bone can be palpated approximately 4 cm above the genitalia (Fig. 2.2). This is the anterior brim of the true pelvis. This ridge is depressed centrally

where the two pubic bones join (the pubic [*pubes* (L) = the growth of hair in the region in adulthood] symphysis) and is marked superiorly on either side by the **pubic tubercles**. These are both palpable, approximately 1 cm on either side of the midline on the upper border of the pubis. This area is quite tender on palpation and is frequently covered with a fatty pad of tissue which may make positive identification of these tubercles difficult. Laterally, the superior ramus of the pubis can be palpated, gradually becoming hidden by muscle.

If the line of the pubic crest is extended laterally beyond the region of the hip joint to the lateral aspect of the upper thigh, a hard, bony prominence can be palpated; this is the **greater trochanter of the femur** (Fig. 2.2). It lies approximately 10 cm below the most lateral aspect of the iliac crest. The trochanters are quadrilateral in shape and, although surrounded by muscle, are easy to identify, being the most lateral bony part of the hip region. This tends to be the level around which the measurement of the hip circumference is erroneously taken.

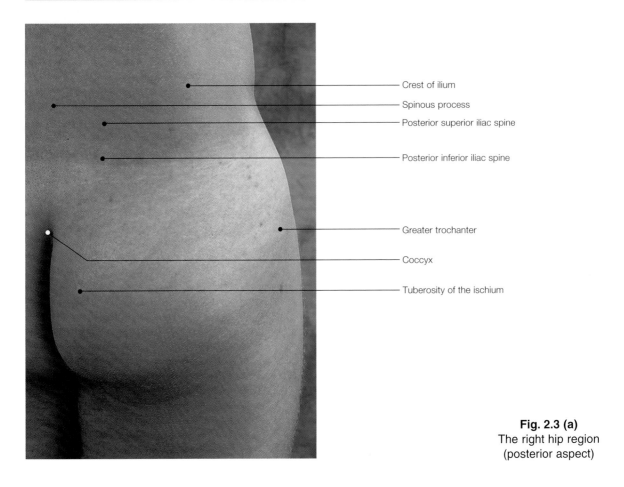

Crest of ilium

Spinous process

Posterior superior iliac spine

Posterior inferior iliac spine

Greater trochanter

Coccyx

Tuberosity of the ischium

Fig. 2.3 (a)
The right hip region
(posterior aspect)

From the back, the ease of palpation depends to a large extent on the build of the subject. The region is often covered with a thick layer of fat, particularly in women, rendering precise identification of bony points extremely difficult.

Returning to the **iliac crest**, it can be traced backwards and medially until the PSIS is reached (Fig. 2.3). This is, however, less easy to identify than the ASIS. In women, it is often located in a small dimple characteristic of this region. From the PSIS the posterior border passes downwards and slightly medially, being concave posteriorly, to terminate approximately 2.5 cm below at the **posterior inferior iliac spine** (PIIS). From here the posterior border passes forwards, forming the upper boundary of the greater sciatic notch. The notch itself is difficult to identify, except in lean subjects.

The lower lateral border of the sacrum [*sacer* (L) = sacred; this is believed to be due to it being the only bone to survive a sacrifice] (S4,5) forms the medial component of the sciatic notch. It can easily be identified running downwards and medially to the cleft between the buttocks and terminating at the coccyx, which is often tucked forwards towards the anal canal. The upper part of the sacrum is held between the two ilia posteriorly, its upper border being on a line 2 cm above the level of the PSIS. If you run your hand down the centre of the sacrum posteriorly, a series of up to five tubercles, gradually diminishing in size, can be felt. These lie in line with the spines of the lumbar vertebrae and are termed **spinous processes** (Fig. 2.3). On either side of these spines, smaller tubercles can be palpated, in line with the articular processes of the vertebrae above. These are therefore known as the articular tubercles. This area is often covered with a fatty pad of tissue which may make positive identification of these tubercles difficult.

The **ischial** [*ischion* (Gk) = the socket in which the thigh bone turns] **tuberosity** is palpable in the standing or prone lying position, being anterolateral to the lateral border of the sacrum and posteromedial to the **greater trochanter** of the femur (Fig. 2.3). It is much easier, however, to identify these tuberosities if the subject either sits on your hands or is in the prone kneeling position. When sitting, large rounded processes can be felt carrying most of the weight of the trunk to the supporting surface. If the subject is asked

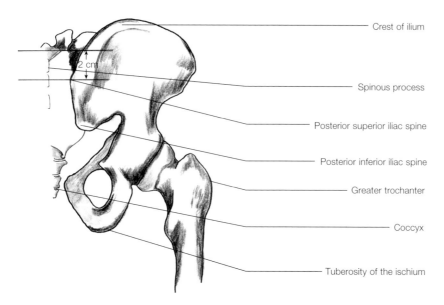

Crest of ilium

2 cm

Spinous process

Posterior superior iliac spine

Posterior inferior iliac spine

Greater trochanter

Coccyx

Tuberosity of the ischium

Fig. 2.3 (b)
Bones of the right hip region
(posterior aspect)

to move gently from side to side, the transference of weight from one tuberosity to the other can be observed. In sustained sitting on a hard surface, such as a wooden pew, these tuberosities become very tender and uncomfortable. The pressure is increased if the subject sits upright, preventing his or her sacrum sliding forward to take some of the weight. The lower area of the tuberosities are covered partially by a bursa medially, and the tendinous attachment of the adductor magnus laterally. The bursa may become inflamed after long periods of sitting upright, causing acute pain over the area (bursitis).

Palpation on movement

Once the position and shape of the pelvis has been established by palpation it is useful to know how its position may change during movements. One can normally consider the bony pelvis, i.e. the two hip bones and the sacrum, as one unit which moves as a whole.

Stand on the right side of the standing model and place your right hand on the upper anterior part of the ilium, place your left hand on the sacrum. If the model now drops the lower abdomen forwards by arching the lumbar spine the pelvis will be observed tilting forwards. If the model now pulls in the lower abdomen and flattens the lumbar spine the pelvis will be observed tilting backwards. Both movements occur around a frontal axis running through the heads of both femora.

Now stand facing the model, who is standing on one leg (the right). Place one hand on the crest of both ilia. The model can now draw up the left side of the pelvis by using the left trunk side flexors of the same side and the hip abductors of the standing leg. If these muscles are relaxed the pelvis will drop on the left side. This lateral tilting of the pelvis occurs around a sagittal axis through the right hip joint. Repeat the same procedure using the left leg as the standing leg.

Stand behind the standing model and place your fingers over the two greater trochanters. If the model flexes and extends the right hip rhythmically the trochanter will be observed rotating anticlockwise on flexion and clockwise on extension.

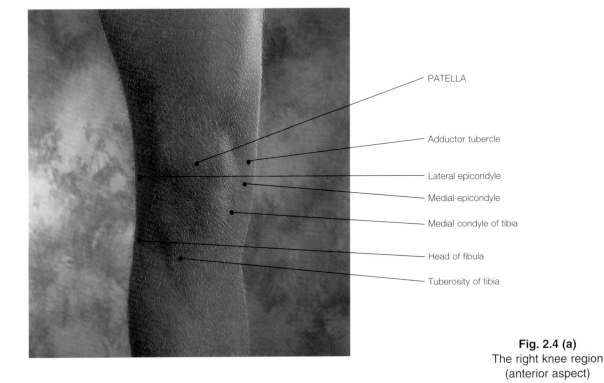

PATELLA

Adductor tubercle

Lateral epicondyle

Medial epicondyle

Medial condyle of tibia

Head of fibula

Tuberosity of tibia

Fig. 2.4 (a)
The right knee region
(anterior aspect)

THE KNEE REGION

There are four bones that can be palpated in this region: the **femur**, the **tibia**, the **fibula** and the **patella**.

The femur [*femur* (L) = a thigh] is the longest and strongest bone in the human body, taking the weight from the hip and transferring it through the knee joint to the tibia. This beautifully shaped bone narrows in its middle half, becoming more or less cylindrical with a very broad posterior border, the linea aspera. It broadens in its lower half, forming two large condyles at its lower end. These project backwards, being separated from each other by the intercondylar notch. The lateral condyle is stouter than the medial, which is slightly longer from front to back. Both condyles are smooth on their posterior, inferior and anterior surfaces, covered by hyaline cartilage in the living body. The smooth surfaces meet anteriorly at a triangular, patella, surface. The lateral surface of the lateral condyle is roughened and is marked just below its centre by a tubercle termed the **lateral epicondyle**. The medial condyle is also roughened on its medial side and marked just below its centre by a slightly larger tubercle termed the **medial epicondyle**. Each condyle has a sharp border above termed the medial and lateral supracondylar ridges, the medial presenting a tubercle at its lower end, the **adductor tubercle**.

The tibia [*tibia* (L) = a flute] is again a very strong stout bone carrying the body weight to the ankle joint and foot. It is broader above, having two large condyles, both flattened superiorly, being slightly depressed centrally. They are separated by the intercondylar eminence and a roughened area anteriorly and posteriorly. The shaft narrows as it descends, presenting a large tubercle anteriorly, the tibial tuberosity, just below the level of the knee joint. The sharp anterior border (shin) passes vertically down from this tubercle.

The patella [*patella* (L) = a small plate] is, as its name implies, a small flat bone situated on the front of the knee. It is triangular in shape with the apex downwards and has a roughened anterior surface and a smooth posterior surface divided into two articular facets with the roughened apex below.

The fibula [*fibula* (L) = a pin] is a long, thin bone situated lateral to the tibia, having complex surfaces and a border mainly produced by the muscles attaching to it. It is expanded above and below: the upper expansion, the head, articulates with the undersurface of the lateral condyle of the tibia and takes no part in the knee joint. The lower expansion forms the lateral malleolus and takes part in the formation of the ankle joint.

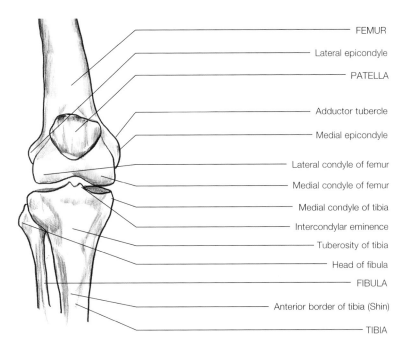

Fig. 2.4 (b)
Bones of the right knee region
(anterior aspect)

Anterior aspect

Palpation

The obvious bony feature anteriorly is the patella. Place your fingers on its anterior surface and gently move them around, investigating its surfaces and borders. The patella is broader superiorly, narrowing to a rounded point below, where it is continuous with the ligamentum patellae. The borders are rounded, while the anterior surface, although appearing slippery due to the presence of the prepatellar bursa, has rough vertical ridges in line with the fibres of the tendon of quadriceps femoris.

With the knee flexed to 90°, the patella becomes more prominent, situated on the medial and lateral femoral condyles, each of which is clearly palpable either side. Each femoral condyle is convex forwards, and presents a strip either side of the patella. It is narrow superiorly, due to the breadth of the patella, but becomes broader below due to the comparative narrowness of the ligamentum patellae. These condylar surfaces pass posteriorly into the knee joint itself.

The medial and lateral tibial condyles are easily recognizable below the femoral condyles, with their flattened upper surfaces being marked by a sharp circumference separating them from the more vertical surfaces of the shaft.

Below and centrally the large tibial tuberosity is easily identified (Fig. 2.4); the lower part is smooth and slippery, due to the presence of the superficial infrapatellar bursa, while its upper part gives attachment to the ligamentum patellae. The tuberosity is particularly noticeable when the knee is extended. With the knee flexed to 90° place your fingers in the small triangular fossae on either side of the ligamentum patellae. Here the upper surfaces of the tibial condyles can be felt below, the under-surface of the femoral condyles above, while between your fingers lies the ligamentum patellae. Directly posteriorly is the cleft of the knee joint, with the medial and lateral menisci between. These are not always palpable, although the anterior edge of the medial meniscus can be observed bulging forwards on medial rotation of the tibia. The anterior edge of the lateral meniscus also becomes palpable, but to a lesser extent, on lateral tibial rotation.

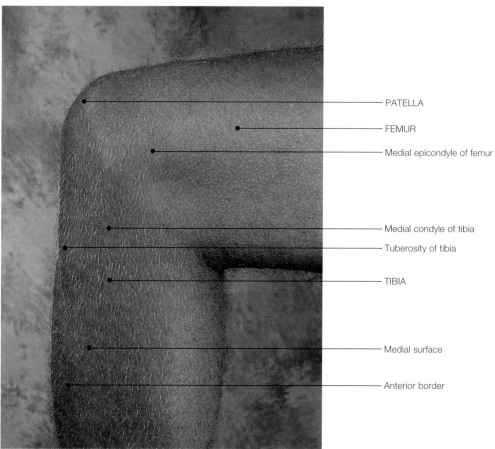

PATELLA

FEMUR

Medial epicondyle of femur

Medial condyle of tibia

Tuberosity of tibia

TIBIA

Medial surface

Anterior border

Fig. 2.4 (c)
The right knee
(medial aspect)

Medial aspect

On the medial side of this region the large, elongated medial condyle of the femur sits on top of the flattened plateau of the medial tibial condyle. The centre of the medial surface of the femoral condyle is marked by a tubercle termed the medial epicondyle. Vertically above this is the medial supracondylar line marked at its lower end by the adductor tubercle.

Below the femoral condyle the flattened **medial tibial condyle** continues downwards as the **medial surface** of the tibial shaft, bounded in front by its **anterior border** marked at its upper end by the **tibial tuberosity**.

Palpation

The medial surface of the femoral condyle is readily palpable, with the epicondyle projecting from its midpoint (Fig. 2.4). Approximately 2 cm proximal to the medial epicondyle the adductor tubercle is just palpable, being hidden to a certain extent by the attachment of the tendinous part of the adductor magnus. This tubercle represents the most distal part of the medial supracondylar ridge, little of which can be palpated.

The medial tibial condyle (Fig. 2.4c,d) is also easily palpable below the femoral condyle. It appears to be larger than the lateral, and can be traced around the medial side, becoming continuous below with the

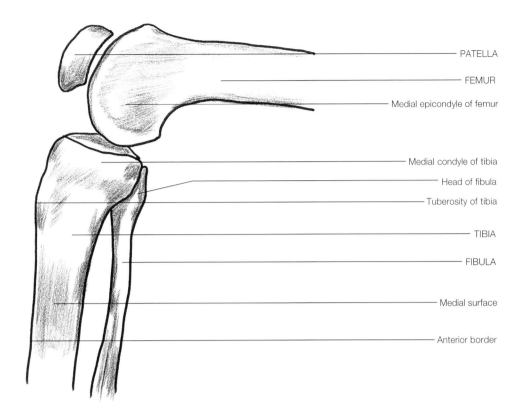

— PATELLA

— FEMUR

— Medial epicondyle of femur

— Medial condyle of tibia

— Head of fibula

— Tuberosity of tibia

— TIBIA

— FIBULA

— Medial surface

— Anterior border

Fig. 2.4 (d)
Bones of the right knee
(medial aspect)

medial surface of the shaft of the tibia and its anterior border (the shin), the whole of which is subcutaneous and palpable as far as the medial malleolus.

Palpation on movement

With the model standing and the knee extended place the fingers of one hand on the medial condyle of the femur and the fingers of the other hand on the medial border of the patella. If the model now flexes the knee the patella will be observed sliding downwards and backwards on the femoral condyle until it lies inferiorly. Return the knee to the extended position. Now move the fingers from the patella and place them on the upper part of the medial surface of the medial condyle of the tibia, close to the joint line. If the knee is flexed again the tibial condyle will be observed moving backwards and upwards onto the posterior aspect of the femoral condyle. As in the case of the lateral condyles, in this position the anterior part of the tibial condyle appears to part from the femoral condyle due to the smaller articular surface at the posterior part of the femoral condyle.

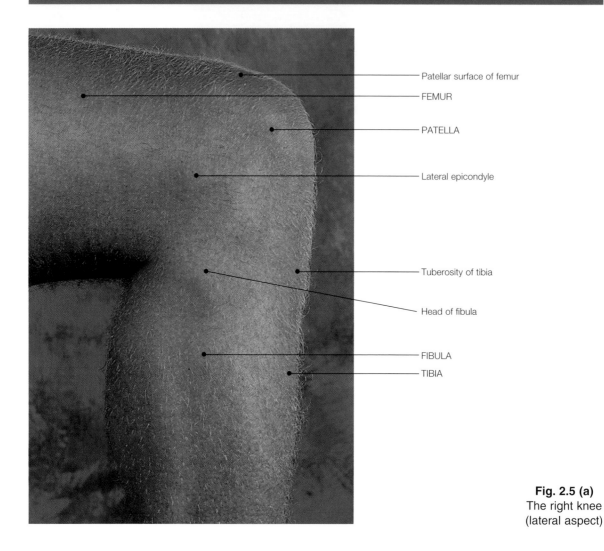

Patellar surface of femur
FEMUR
PATELLA
Lateral epicondyle
Tuberosity of tibia
Head of fibula
FIBULA
TIBIA

Fig. 2.5 (a)
The right knee
(lateral aspect)

Lateral aspect

On the lateral side of this region the stout lateral condyle of the femur sits on top of the plateau of the lateral condyle of the tibia. Posteriorly, the two condyles are close together; however anteriorly, they diverge into a small hollow which is bounded at the front by the lower section of the **patella** and the ligamentum patellae. The **head of the fibula** lies below and posterior to the knee joint.

Palpation

With the model standing, the flat lateral surface of the lateral femoral condyle can readily be palpated, lying posterior to the lateral border of the patella. It is marked by a tubercle at its centre (the lateral epicondyle). Running your fingers upwards from this **lateral epicondyle** the lateral supracondylar ridge may be just palpable running vertically upwards. This is difficult to palpate as the iliotibial tract tends to follow the same line.

Approximately 2 cm below the lateral epicondyle the lower border of the lateral femoral condyle and the upper border of the lateral tibial condyle can be palpated running horizontally and diverging anteriorly. Finally, approximately 1 cm below this rim, the head of the fibula can be palpated, with its styloid process projecting upwards, and the narrower neck just below (Fig. 2.5). The remainder of the upper end

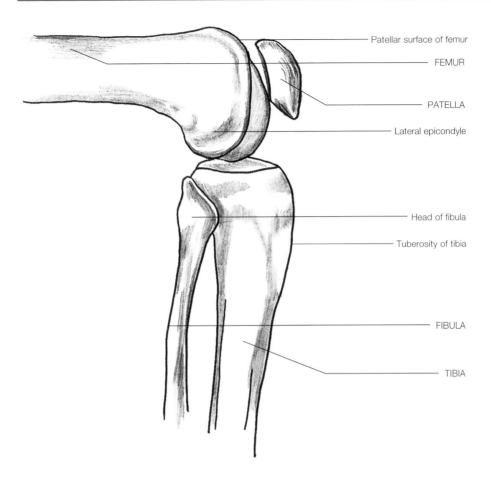

Patellar surface of femur

FEMUR

PATELLA

Lateral epicondyle

Head of fibula

Tuberosity of tibia

FIBULA

TIBIA

Fig. 2.5 (b)
Bones of the right knee
(lateral aspect)

of the shaft of the fibula is surrounded by muscles and is therefore not palpable. The head can easily be located by running the palm of the hand up the lateral aspect of the leg.

Palpation on movement

With the model's knee fully extended, place your fingers of one hand on the lateral side of the patella and the fingers of the other hand on the lateral surface of the femoral condyle. If the model now flexes the knee the patella will be observed sliding downwards and backwards under the condyle, finally ending up inferiorly. Return the knee back to the extended position. Now remove the fingers from the patella and place them on the lateral condyle of the tibia close to the knee joint. If the model flexes the knee again the tibia will be observed gliding backwards and upwards onto the posterior surface of the femoral condyles. At this position the anterior part of the tibial condyle appears to part from the femoral condyle. This is due to the posterior surface of the femoral condyle being smaller than that of the tibia.

The head of the fibula moves with the tibia.

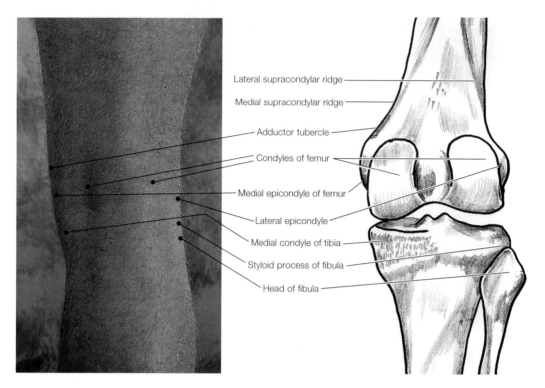

Fig. 2.5 (c), (d)
The right knee region (posterior aspect)

Lateral supracondylar ridge
Medial supracondylar ridge
Adductor tubercle
Condyles of femur
Medial epicondyle of femur
Lateral epicondyle
Medial condyle of tibia
Styloid process of fibula
Head of fibula

Posterior aspect

Virtually no bony features can be palpated on the posterior aspect of the knee, either when it is flexed or extended. The posterior aspect of the sides of each **femoral condyle** and the medial surfaces of the tibia soon become hidden by the fascia and muscles at the back of the knee. The **head of the fibula** (Fig. 2.5), however, can easily be palpated on the lateral side of the popliteal fossa, with the tendon of biceps femoris attaching to its upper section. Palpation from this aspect must be approached with care, as the common peroneal nerve passes down the back of the head of the fibula en route to its passage around the lateral side of the neck.

When the knee is extended and the quadriceps femoris is relaxed, the patella can easily be moved from side to side, producing a knocking effect as it crosses either side of the grooved patellar surface of the femur. This manoeuvre, an accessory movement, exposes a strip of the patellar surface of the femur, on the side away from the direction of the movement. If held to one side, the articular surface of the patella on that side can also be palpated for approximately 1 cm on its posterior surface.

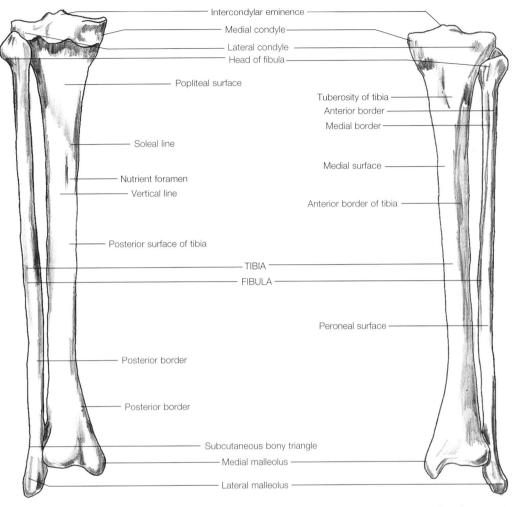

Intercondylar eminence

Medial condyle

Lateral condyle

Head of fibula

Popliteal surface

Tuberosity of tibia

Anterior border

Medial border

Medial surface

Soleal line

Anterior border of tibia

Nutrient foramen

Vertical line

Posterior surface of tibia

TIBIA

FIBULA

Peroneal surface

Posterior border

Posterior border

Subcutaneous bony triangle

Medial malleolus

Lateral malleolus

Posterior aspect

Anterior aspect

Fig. 2.5 (e), (f)
The tibia and fibula

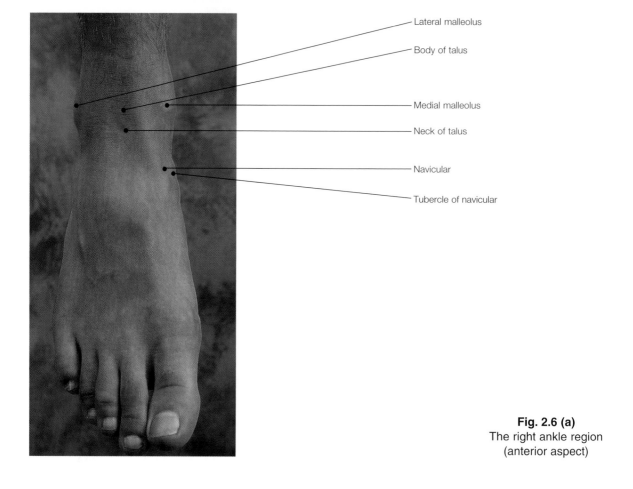

Lateral malleolus

Body of talus

Medial malleolus

Neck of talus

Navicular

Tubercle of navicular

Fig. 2.6 (a)
The right ankle region
(anterior aspect)

THE ANKLE REGION

There are four bones taking part in the formation of this area: the lower ends of the **tibia** and **fibula**, the **talus** and the **calcaneus**.

The lower end of the tibia

From its narrowest cross-section, two-thirds of the way down the shaft, the bone expands to form part of the mortice for the formation of the ankle joint. Its medial side presents a large projection downwards, termed the **medial malleolus**. On its lateral side there is an elongated triangular area for the attachment of an extremely strong interosseous ligament which binds the two bones together. Its under-surface and the lateral side of the malleolus are smooth for articulation with the talus in the ankle joint.

The lower end of the fibula

The slender shaft of the fibula expands below to form the pointed **lateral malleolus**, which forms the lateral section of the mortice of the ankle joint. It is flattened from side to side, having a smooth articular surface on its medial side and a roughened surface on its lateral, subcutaneous side.

The talus

This bone is formed of a **body**, a **neck** and a head. The body is narrower at the back and wider anteriorly. It is pulley-shaped superiorly and slightly concave inferiorly. It has smooth, articular surfaces on its superior, inferior, lateral and the upper part of its medial surfaces.

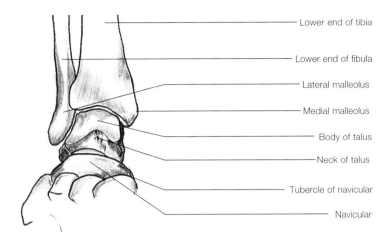

- Lower end of tibia
- Lower end of fibula
- Lateral malleolus
- Medial malleolus
- Body of talus
- Neck of talus
- Tubercle of navicular
- Navicular

Fig. 2.6 (b)
Bones of the right ankle region
(anterior aspect)

The neck passes forwards and medially to expand into the head, which articulates with the posterior surface of the navicular.

The calcaneus (see page 34)

At the ankle the muscles of the leg have become tendinous and thus the bones are easier to palpate and identify between and deep to the tendons and retinacula.

Palpation

Anterior aspect. Placing the hands on the subcutaneous medial surface of the tibia, trace down to the medial malleolus. The anterior border of the tibia (shin) appears to form the anterior part of the malleolus, which is clearly defined (Fig. 2.6a,b). It has an anterior border and tip which can be palpated, and a posterior border which is partially hidden by tendons and the flexor retinaculum. The anterior border of the malleolus [*malleolus* (L) = a small hammer] continues upwards and laterally under the extensor tendons and extensor retinacula, marking the line of the ankle joint.

On the lateral side of the ankle the lateral malleolus of the fibula is the most outstanding feature (Figs 2.5e,f, 2.6). From its tip, which lies at a lower level than that of the medial malleolus, both the anterior and posterior borders can be traced upwards, encompassing the large prominence of the malleolus. Just above the level of the ankle joint, at approximately 2.5 cm, the fibula narrows to a triangular subcutaneous lateral surface. The shaft can be traced upwards for approximately 15 cm, where it becomes hidden by muscle, the peroneus tertius anteriorly and the peroneus brevis and tendon of peroneus longus posteriorly.

With your right hand over the front of the ankle region, place your index finger on the lateral, and your thumb on the medial, malleolus of the subject's left ankle. Draw your finger and thumb forward into a small hollow on either side. Between your thumb and finger you will feel the head of the talus. Immediately anterior you can palpate the narrow gap of the talonavicular joint and posterior part of the navicular with its prominent **tubercle**, medially. If the foot is plantar flexed, the neck of the talus [*talus* (L) = the ankle bone] can also be palpated, and deep beneath the tip of your index finger, just lateral to the head of the talus, you will feel the anterior section of the upper surface of the calcaneus [*calx* (L) = a heel] and the origin of extensor digitorum brevis.

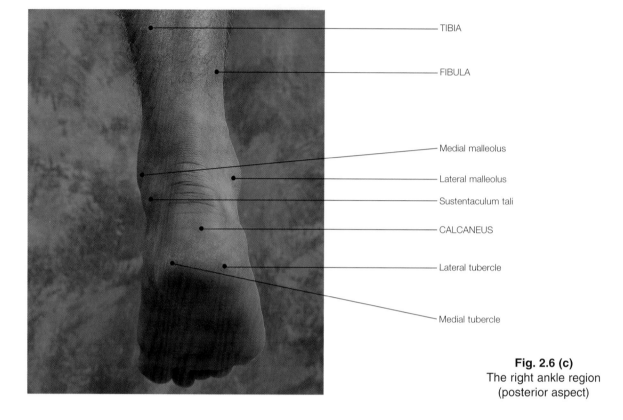

TIBIA

FIBULA

Medial malleolus

Lateral malleolus

Sustentaculum tali

CALCANEUS

Lateral tubercle

Medial tubercle

Fig. 2.6 (c)
The right ankle region
(posterior aspect)

Posterior aspect. From the posterior aspect very little of the talus can be seen as the body has narrowed down to just two tubercles and a groove running downwards and medially. The mortice of the ankle joint (see page 32) is formed by the two malleoli and the inferior border of the tibia. Both the malleoli are marked posteriorly by a fossa for the attachment of ligaments.

THE CALCANEUS

This is the largest of the tarsal bones and is situated below the talus and behind the navicular and cuboid. It is oblong in shape, projecting forwards and backwards beyond the talus. The backward projection forms the heel. It has six surfaces: an anterior, which is smooth, a superior, marked by a smooth articular surface centrally, and a medial, which is fairly smooth and converted into a hollow by the projection medially from its upper section by the sustentaculum tali. The lateral surface is roughened, presenting two tubercles, and the posterior surface is rounded and roughened across its centre for the attachment of the tendo calcaneus. Its inferior surface is slightly concave downwards and is roughened for the attachment of muscles and fascia. It presents three broad, rounded

tubercles. The medial and lateral lie posterior, almost on the junction with the posterior surface, and the anterior lies central, approximately 1 cm from its anterior border.

Palpation

Place your hands at the tip of the medial malleolus. Move your fingers 1 cm down from this tip and you will feel the horizontal ridge of the sustentaculum tali. It runs for approximately 2–3 cm and is clearer anteriorly and posteriorly. If the foot is everted the sustentaculum tali becomes more prominent. At the anterior end of this ridge there is a small gap before encountering the tubercle of the navicular. This gap is spanned by the 'spring ligament'.

Because the tendo calcaneus lies almost 2 cm clear of the ankle joint, few bony features can be identified posteriorly. On close examination of the posterior borders of the lateral and medial malleoli, a small depression can be palpated, the malleolar fossa. Tracing superiorly, the posterior border of the lateral malleolus forms the posterior border of the triangular area referred to above. The posterior surface of the medial malleolus is continuous with the posterior border of the medial surface of the tibia (Fig. 2.6c,d).

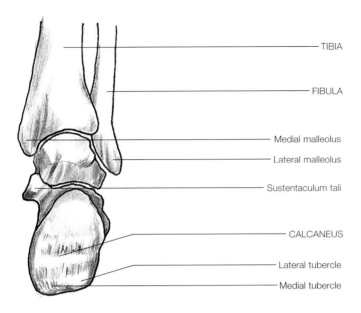

Fig. 2.6 (d)
Bones of the right ankle region
(posterior aspect)

Palpation on movement

Anterior. With the model lying, stand facing the lateral side of the model's right ankle region. With your left hand grip the two malleoli with your fingers on the medial and your thumb on the lateral. With your right hand grip the anterior part of the body and neck of the talus with your fingers in the hollow just anterior to the medial malleolus and your thumb in the hollow just anterior to the lateral malleolus. Both sets of fingers and both thumbs should be close to each other.

Starting from the fully plantarflexed position, if the model now dorsiflexes the foot you will feel the anterior part of the body disappearing into the gap between the two malleoli. In fact, the fingers of your right hand will now be gripping the neck and head of the talus. At this point the ankle is in its close-packed position and no side-to-side movement is possible. When the model fully plantarflexes from the dorsiflexed position the head and neck of the talus will move forwards and downwards and the anterior section of the body will reappear from within the mortice. At this point the head and neck of the talus can be rocked from side to side. This is an accessory movement.

Medial. With the ankle returned to the midposition, adopt the same position with your hands but now move the fingers of your right hand to just below the tip of the medial malleolus. Here you will find the horizontal rim of the sustentaculum tali. If the model now rhythmically plantar- and dorsiflexes the ankle, you will feel the sustentaculum tali moving forwards and backwards, describing a shallow arc around the medial malleolus.

Lateral. Similarly, if the left hand remains in its original position and your right thumb is placed on the two tubercles below the lateral malleolus, movement forwards and backwards around the malleolus can be observed when plantar- and dorsiflexion is performed.

Posterior. With the model and yourself in the same position, keep your left hand gripping the two malleoli, place your right hand under the heel with the fingers resting on the posterior aspect of the calcaneus either side of the tendo calcaneus. As the model moves into dorsi- and plantarflexion, the calcaneus will be observed moving forwards and backwards away and towards the posterior part of the tibia. It is worth noting that when it passes downwards it is nearly impossible to move from side to side. This is due to the anterior part of the talus moving into the mortice of the ankle joint.

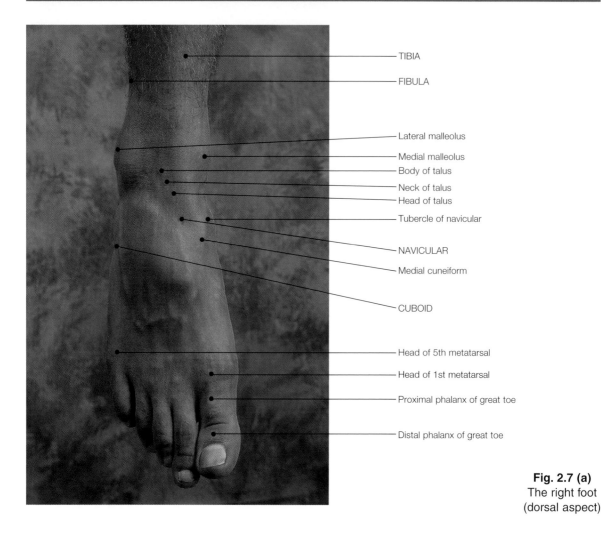

TIBIA

FIBULA

Lateral malleolus

Medial malleolus
Body of talus
Neck of talus
Head of talus
Tubercle of navicular

NAVICULAR
Medial cuneiform

CUBOID

Head of 5th metatarsal

Head of 1st metatarsal

Proximal phalanx of great toe

Distal phalanx of great toe

Fig. 2.7 (a)
The right foot
(dorsal aspect)

THE FOOT

There are three main groups of bones forming the skeleton of the foot. Posteriorly is the tarsus, comprising large irregular bones, while anteriorly are the phalanges, miniature long bones forming the toes. Between these two groups are the metatarsals, which are also miniature long bones, linking them together (Fig. 2.7).

The calcaneus forms the heel and is the largest and most posterior of the group of tarsal bones. In front and to the lateral side is the **cuboid** [*kubgides* (Gk) = cube shape]. Sitting on the middle section of the upper surface of the calcaneus is the **body of the talus**, with its **neck and head** passing forwards and medially, superomedially to the cuboid. The **navicular** lies in front of the head of the talus with the three cuneiform [*cuneus* (L) = a wedge] bones interposed between the anterior surface of the navicular and the three medial

metatarsal bones. The two lateral metatarsals lie anterior to the cuboid.

Dorsal aspect

From the medial and lateral malleoli run your index finger and thumb forwards, as before, until the head of the talus is gripped between them. The upper part of the talocalcaneonavicular joint can be palpated. The roughened dorsal surface of the navicular can be traced medially to its large tuberosity which projects downwards and medially, being approximately 2.5 cm downwards and forwards from the tip of the medial malleolus (Figs 2.6a,b, and 2.7). Immediately distal to the navicular the **medial cuneiform** can also be palpated, projecting downwards. The dorsal surfaces of

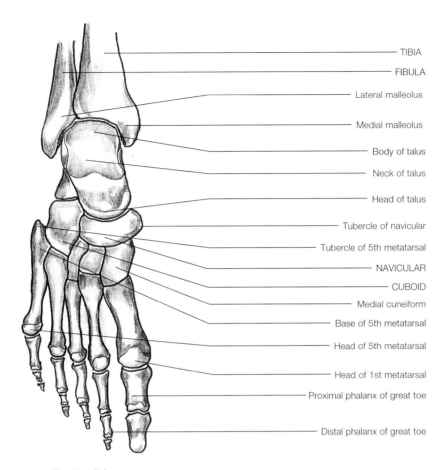

TIBIA
FIBULA
Lateral malleolus
Medial malleolus
Body of talus
Neck of talus
Head of talus
Tubercle of navicular
Tubercle of 5th metatarsal
NAVICULAR
CUBOID
Medial cuneiform
Base of 5th metatarsal
Head of 5th metatarsal
Head of 1st metatarsal
Proximal phalanx of great toe
Distal phalanx of great toe

Fig. 2.7 (b)
Bones of the right foot
(dorsal aspect)

the middle and lateral cuneiforms can be identified on the dorsum of the foot, lying lateral to the medial cuneiform. The base, shaft and **head of the first metatarsal** are clearly identifiable, being much stouter than those of the other four. In some individuals the head projects medially, carrying the base of the toe with it. This causes inflammation of the bursa on its medial side, often accompanied by pain and swelling. Such medial deviation of the metatarsal head commonly progresses to a condition termed 'hallux valgus'.

Carefully running the pads of your fingers over the dorsum of the foot, the base, shaft and head of each of the remaining metatarsals can be palpated. The base of the second metatarsal is traced further proximally than the others to the middle cuneiform, the third to the lateral cuneiform and the fourth and fifth to the cuboid (Fig. 2.7). The **base of the fifth metatarsal** is more expanded than the rest and has, projecting proximally, a **tubercle or styloid process** on its lateral side. The base is easily located by tracing backwards along the shaft of the fifth metatarsal. The large lateral projection is elongated proximally and overlies the lateral side of the cuboid.

The lateral side of the calcaneus is marked by the peroneal tubercle 1 cm below and just anterior to the tip of the lateral malleolus. This tubercle is elongated downwards and forwards and if the foot is everted, two tendons appear to pull clear. The one above the tubercle is peroneus brevis, the one below is peroneus longus. This tubercle must not be confused with that of the calcaneofibular ligament which can be found with careful palpation just below and posterior to the tip of the lateral malleolus.

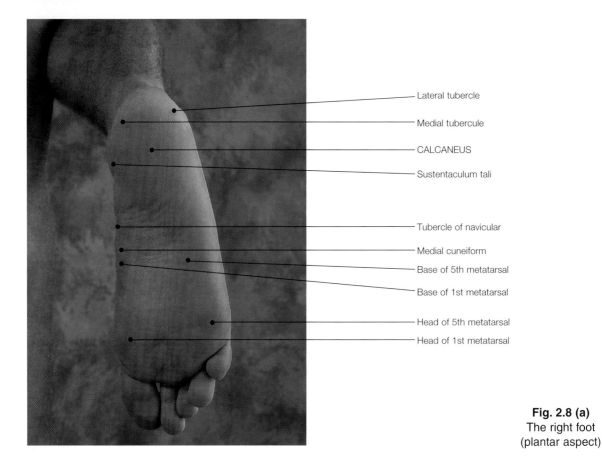

- Lateral tubercle
- Medial tubercule
- CALCANEUS
- Sustentaculum tali
- Tubercle of navicular
- Medial cuneiform
- Base of 5th metatarsal
- Base of 1st metatarsal
- Head of 5th metatarsal
- Head of 1st metatarsal

Fig. 2.8 (a)
The right foot
(plantar aspect)

Plantar aspect

Very few bony points are palpable in this region due to the presence of overlying muscles, as well as a dense and thick layer of plantar fascia, termed the 'plantar aponeurosis'.

The heel is the most posterior and inferior aspect of the **calcaneus**, on either side of which are two large broad **tubercles** (**medial** and **lateral**) which give attachment to the more superficial of the plantar muscles. On the posterior aspect of the heel there is often a horizontal raised area to which the tendo calcaneus attaches. The tendon and its attachment are usually quite clear (see Fig. 4.5b). Below this the posterior surface of the calcaneus is covered with a pad of tough fibrous tissue and fat.

Below and in front of the tip of the lateral malleolus, the calcaneus is marked by an elongated tubercle (the peroneal tubercle), which has the tendons of peroneus brevis above and peroneus longus below.

Immediately below the tip of the medial malleolus, a horizontal ridge can be felt – the sustentaculum tali – which is slightly hidden by the tendon of flexor digitorum longus. The inferior surface of the navicular tuberosity can be palpated on the medial side of the foot 3 cm anteroinferior to the tip of the medial malleolus. On the lateral side of the foot, the base of the fifth metatarsal and its tubercle are covered by the plantar fascia and muscles. The **heads** of the metatarsals are relatively easy to find (Fig. 2.8). If the toe is grasped between the finger and thumb of one hand and passively extended, the metatarsal head can readily be felt on the plantar surface proximal to the base of the toe. If, however, the toe is flexed at the metatarsophalangeal joint, the metatarsal head appears on the dorsum of the foot, as the knuckles would in the hand.

The base of the proximal phalanx can be identified just beyond the corresponding metatarsal head. The heads of the proximal phalanges, particularly those of the second, third and fourth, are often flexed and project forwards on their dorsum, being covered by hard skin and a bursa which often swells and becomes inflamed, a condition known as 'hammer toes'. If the toes are extended at the proximal interphalangeal joint, the small bicondylar head can be identified (Fig. 2.8).

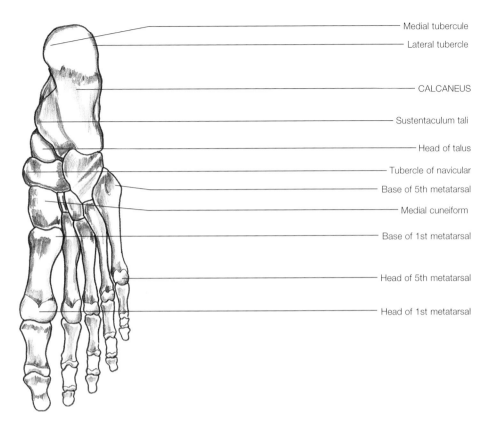

Medial tubercule

Lateral tubercle

CALCANEUS

Sustentaculum tali

Head of talus

Tubercle of navicular

Base of 5th metatarsal

Medial cuneiform

Base of 1st metatarsal

Head of 5th metatarsal

Head of 1st metatarsal

Fig. 2.8 (b)
Bones of the right foot
(plantar aspect)

Palpation on movement

Take up the same position and the same hand holds as for palpation on movement, anterior aspect (page 35). If the model now plantarflexes the ankle and then moves the foot into adduction and abduction, the **head of the talus** can be observed moving from side to side. Remember, this will not occur in dorsiflexion due to the close-packed nature of the ankle joint.

Now move your hands down so that the head of the talus is gripped in the left hand and the right fingers come into contact with the tubercle of the navicular and the thumb grips around the base of the fifth metatarsal. As the model everts the foot, the tubercle will descend and the metatarsal rises. As the model inverts the foot, the tubercle will rise and the metatarsal will descend. The navicular is rotating around an axis running through the neck and head of the talus.

If the hands are now moved down to the base of the great toe and the left hand grips the first metatarsal just proximal to the head and the right hand grips the proximal phalanx, when the model extends the toe, the head becomes quite clear with the phalanx moving towards the dorsum of the head. When the toe is flexed, the phalanx can be palpated moving downwards around the head. This movement can be observed in all the metatarsophalangeal joints, but to a lesser extent.

A similar movement can be felt in the interphalangeal joints with the head of the phalanx becoming quite palpable when the toes are flexed.

SELF-ASSESSMENT QUESTIONS

Page 16

1. Describe the bony boundaries of the thoracic outlet.

2. Give the names and positions of the bones which comprise the pelvic inlet.

3. Which bones form the posterior boundary of the abdomen?

4. The costal angle is formed by which costal cartilage?

5. What forms the lowest extremity of the thoracic outlet?

6. On a level with what part of which vertebra does the tip of the 12th rib lie?

7. Name any other structure which lies on this level.

Page 17

8. Describe the steps involved in locating the anterior superior iliac spine.

9. What bony feature lies on the lateral lip of the crest of the ilium 5 cm posterior to the anterior superior spine?

10. Which bony features are palpable 5 cm above the genitalia?

11. What structure lies centrally at this point?

12. Describe the attachments of both ends of the inguinal ligament.

Page 18

13. How many lumbar vertebrae are found in the vertebral column?

14. Of these vertebrae, which is the largest and which is the smallest?

15. Which lumbar vertebra presents the largest transverse processes?

16. On a typical lumbar vertebra, in which direction do the upper articular processes face?

17. Generally, in which direction do the inferior articular facets face?

18. Identify any exceptions.

Please complete the labels below.

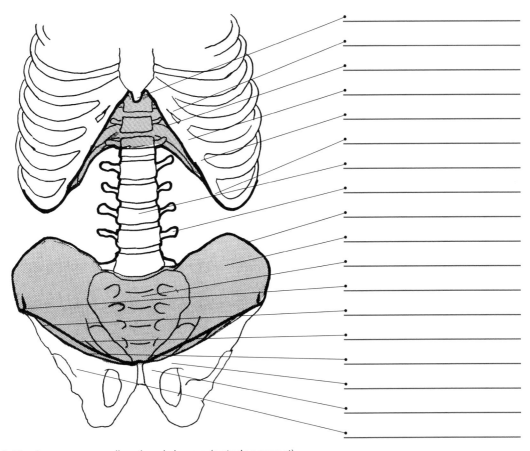

Fig. 2.1 (a) The bones surrounding the abdomen (anterior aspect)

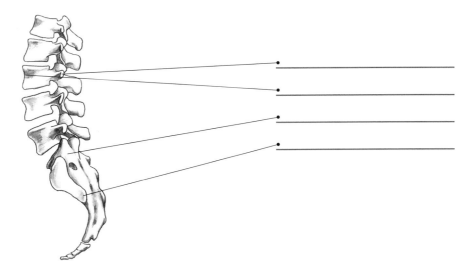

Fig. 2.1 (b) The bones surrounding the abdomen (lateral aspect, viewed from left)

19. Viewed from above, what shape is the neural canal in the lumbar spine?

20. What shape are the lumbar spines posteriorly?

21. Explain why there is a small hollow immediately above the central part of the sacrum.

22. When the spine is flexed, explain why the small gaps between the spines normally disappear.

23. What structure can be palpated 5 cm lateral to the spines?

24. Which muscles make the identification of bony features difficult in this region?

25. Which vertebrae are normally fused to form the sacrum?

26. Describe the shape and position of the sacrum.

27. In which area is there visible evidence of the sacrum being composed of five vertebrae?

28. What bony features lie down the middle of the sacrum's posterior surface?

29. What structure can be palpated on either side of the sacrum?

30. Which bones comprise the lateral mass of the sacrum?

31. With what structure does the lateral mass of the sacrum articulate?

Page 19

32. Between which two bones does the sacrum lie?

33. Which part of the sacrum projects backwards?

34. Name the bone which lies at the lower end of the sacrum.

35. From which bones is this structure formed?

36. Describe the method by which this bone can be palpated.

Please complete the labels below.

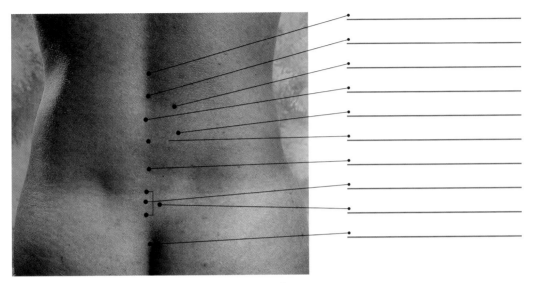

Fig. 2.1 (c) The lumbar vertebrae and sacrum (posterior aspect)

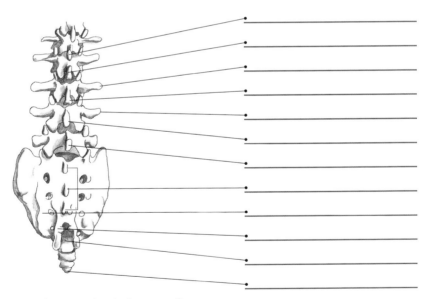

Fig. 2.1 (d) The lumbar vertebrae and sacrum (posterior aspect)

Page 20

37. Which three bones form the pelvic girdle?

38. Describe what is meant by the 'true pelvis'.

39. Explain the term 'false pelvis'.

40. By what Latin name is the hip bone known?

41. List the three components of the hip bone.

42. Where are the three bones united?

43. What forms the upper boundary of the ilium?

44. What structures form the boundaries of the obturator foramen?

45. Which three bony processes form the upper end of the femur?

46. Explain why this area is difficult to palpate.

47. The lower boundary of the waist is limited by which bony landmarks?

Page 21

48. Where is the anterior superior iliac spine located?

49. What lies at the posterior end of the iliac crest?

50. Describe the shape of the iliac crest from above.

51. What lies 5 cm posterior to the ASIS on the lateral side of the crest of the ilium?

52. Which structure attaches to this process?

53. Approximately, how far apart are the two anterior superior iliac spines?

54. Name the bony process which lies approximately 2 cm below the anterior superior iliac spine just above the acetabulum.

55. Name the rim of bone palpable at the lower, central part of the abdomen and approximately 4 cm above the genitalia.

56. What can be palpated centrally on this rim?

Please complete the labels below.

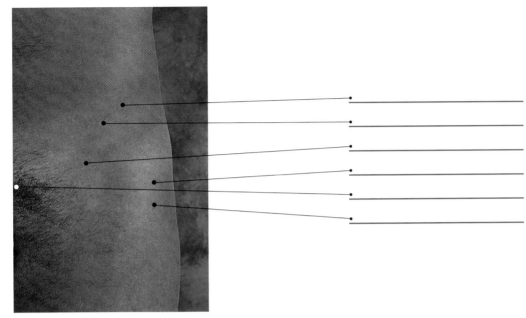

Fig. 2.2 (a) The left hip region (anterior aspect)

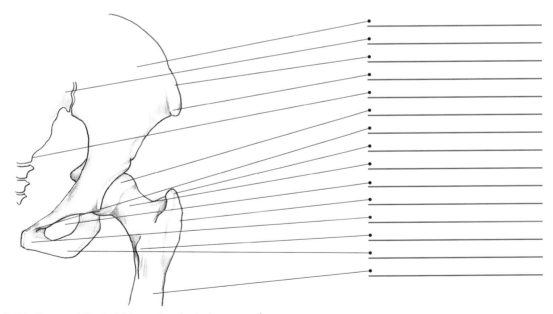

Fig. 2.2 (b) Bones of the left hip region (anterior aspect)

57. List the bones and the processes which comprise this rim.

_____

58. About 10 cm below the iliac crest, laterally, a large bony process is palpable. What is it called?

_____

Page 22

59. Name the process which lies approximately 2.5 cm below the posterior superior iliac spine.

60. What notch does the posterior border partially form below this point?

61. Which bone forms the medial boundary of this notch?

62. Name the bony process at the lower end of the sacrum.

63. How far above the line of the posterior superior iliac spines does the upper border of the sacrum reach?

64. Which bony processes lie centrally down the posterior aspect of the sacrum?

65. What name is given to the line of tubercles which lie just lateral to the midline of the sacrum?

66. Explain why this area is difficult to palpate.

67. What lies at the lower end of the ischium?

68. How is this structure made easier to palpate?

Page 23

69. What partially covers the two tuberosities, posteriorly?

70. The tuberosities give attachment to which muscle tendon?

71. What may occur in these bursii if they are put under pressure for a period of time?

72. If the lumbar spine is arched and the abdomen dropped forward, in which direction does the pelvis rotate?

73. Around which axis does this movement occur?

74. Lateral tilting of the pelvis occurs around which axis?

75. Name the muscle groups which produce this movement.

76. Explain how one can produce forward and backward rotation of the pelvis.

Please complete the labels below.

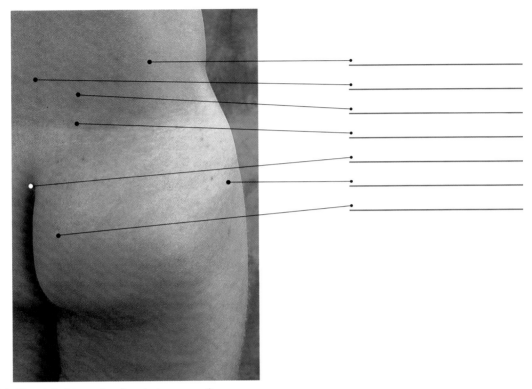

Fig. 2.3 (a) The right hip region (posterior aspect)

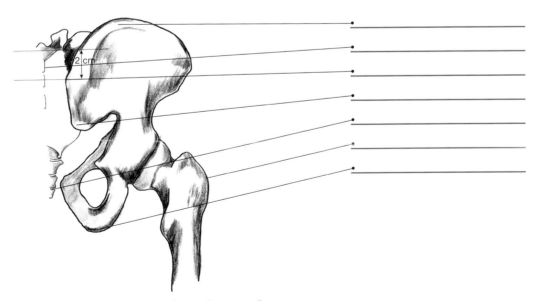

Fig. 2.3 (b) Bones of the right hip region (posterior aspect)

Page 24

77. Which three bones take part in the knee joint?

78. What term is used to describe the posterior border of the femur?

79. Name the notch which lies posteriorly at the lower end of the femur.

80. Which is the stouter of the two femoral condyles?

81. From anterior to posterior, which is the longer condyle?

82. What type of cartilage covers the condyles inferiorly?

83. By what name is the triangular articular surface on the front of the two femoral condyles known?

84. Name the ridge above the two condyles, posteriorly.

85. What is the term used to describe the central raised area between the two condyles of the tibia?

86. What shape is the patella?

87. Which area of the patella is smooth and covered with articular cartilage?

88. With what does the upper end of the fibula articulate?

89. What bony prominence does its lower end form?

90. In which direction does the apex of the patella point?

Page 25

91. What attaches to the base of the patella?

92. The apex of the patella gives attachment to which ligament?

93. What structure covers the lower part of the tuberosity of the tibia?

94. Where may the two menisci be palpated?

Page 26

95. In which area is the medial epicondyle of the femur located?

96. Which tubercle lies just above the medial epicondyle?

97. Name the ridge which runs vertically up from this tubercle.

Please complete the labels below.

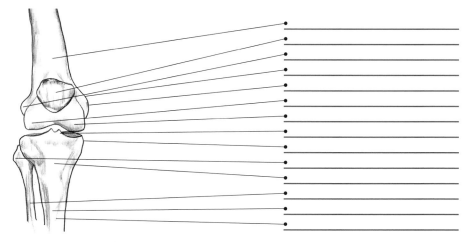

Fig. 2.4 (b) Bones of the right knee region (anterior aspect)

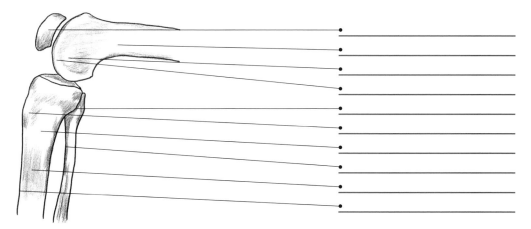

Fig. 2.4 (d) Bones of the right knee (medial aspect)

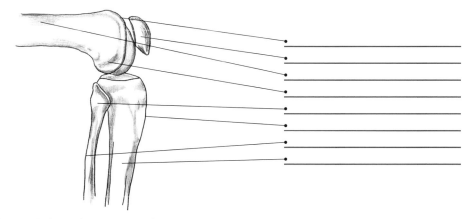

Fig. 2.5 (b) Bones of the right knee (lateral aspect)

98. The flattened medial condyle of the tibia continues downwards as what structure?

99. What structure bounds this surface anteriorly?

100. Of the following three structures, which is the easiest and which is the most difficult to palpate: the medial epicondyle of the femur, the adductor tubercle or the medial supracondylar ridge?

101. How far down the leg is the medial surface of the tibia palpable?

Page 27

102. What is the anterior border of the tibia commonly called?

103. Which tubercle projects laterally from the midpoint of the lateral condyle of the femur?

104. How far below the knee joint is the head of the fibula situated?

105. What projects upwards from the head of the fibula?

Page 28

106. What structure lies below the lateral condyle of the femur?

107. Name the projection of bone which is palpable below the knee joint on the lateral side.

108. What marks the centre of the lateral surface of the lateral condyle of the femur?

109. Explain why it is difficult to palpate the lateral supracondylar ridge.

110. How far below the rim of the lateral condyle of the tibia can the head of the fibula be palpated?

Page 29

111. Explain why it is difficult to palpate the middle sections of the shaft of the fibula.

112. Describe how the head of the fibula may be easily palpated.

113. When the knee is being flexed, in which direction does the patella move?

114. With which part of the femoral condyle is the tibia in contact when the knee is in full flexion?

115. Describe the process which projects upwards from the head of the fibula.

Page 30

116. Which muscle attaches to the head of the fibula either side of this process?

Please complete the labels below.

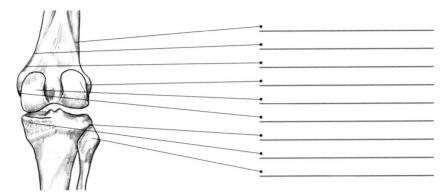

Fig. 2.5 (d) The right knee region (posterior aspect)

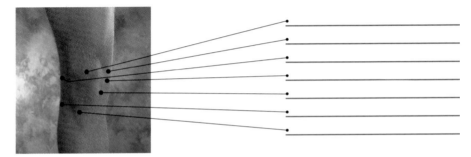

Fig. 2.4 (a) The right knee region (anterior aspect)

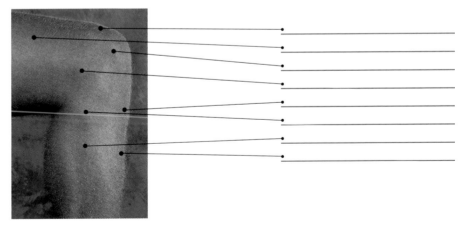

Fig. 2.5 (a) The right knee (lateral aspect)

117. Name a ligament which also attaches to the head of the fibula.

_____

118. Which nerve winds around the neck and back of the head of the fibula?

_____

Page 32

119. What bones take part in the ankle joint?

_____

120. What is the name of the projection downwards at the lower end of the tibia?

_____

121. With what bone does this projection articulate in the ankle joint?

_____

122. List the bony components of the talus.

_____

123. In which direction does the talar neck pass from the body?

_____

124. With which bone does the head of the talus articulate anteriorly?

_____

125. The tip of which malleolus projects the lowest?

_____

126. Which joint can be palpated just anterior to the head of the talus?

_____

127. Describe the posterior surface of the talus.

_____

Page 34

128. Which bones form the mortice of the ankle joint?

_____

129. What attaches to the fossa on the posterior border of the medial malleolus?

_____

130. Name the largest tarsal bone.

_____

131. What structure projects medially from the upper part of the medial surface of the calcaneus?

_____

132. Where does the tendo calcaneus attach to the calcaneus?

_____

133. List the three tubercles on the inferior surface of the calcaneus.

_____

134. How far below the tip of the medial malleolus is the sustentaculum tali?

_____

135. Describe a way in which the sustentaculum tali can be made more prominent.

_____

136. What structure spans the gap between the anterior part of the sustentaculum tali and the navicular bone?

_____

137. By what other name is this structure known?

_____

Page 35

138. Describe what happens to the body of the talus on dorsiflexion of the ankle.

_____

Please complete the labels below.

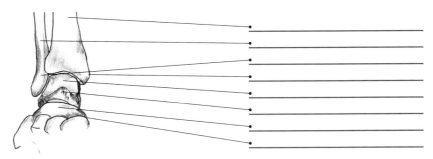

Fig. 2.6 (b) Bones of the right ankle region (anterior aspect)

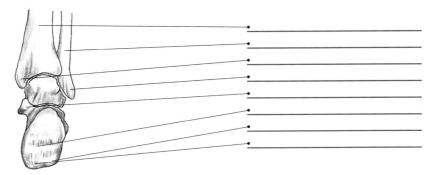

Fig. 2.6 (d) Bones of the right ankle region (posterior aspect)

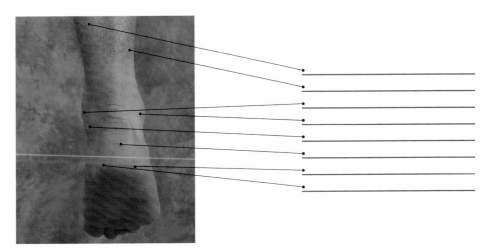

Fig. 2.6 (c) The right ankle region (posterior aspect)

139. How much side to side movement occurs at the ankle joint when it is dorsiflexed?

140. What type of movement does the sustentaculum tali produce on plantar and dorsiflexion of the ankle joint?

Page 36

141. How many groups of bones form the skeleton of the foot?

142. Name these groups, from posterior to anterior.

143. Which bones form the posterior group?

144. What structure projects downwards from the medial aspect of the navicular?

145. How far is this structure from the tip of the medial malleolus?

146. Which bones lie anterior to the navicula?

Page 37

147. In what ways does the first metatarsal bone differ from the other metatarsal bones?

148. Name the condition in which the head of the medial metatarsal projects more medially than normal.

149. Which metatarsal bones articulate with the cuboid bone?

150. List the identifying features of the fifth metatarsal.

151. Name the elongated tubercle, on the lateral surface of the calcaneus, anterior and below the tip of the lateral malleolus.

152. Which two tendons pass above and below this tubercle?

Page 38

153. Which is the upper of these two tendons?

154. Name the thick fascia under the plantar aspect of the foot.

155. What structure covers the posterior inferior aspect of the calcaneus?

156. Which tendon runs over the sustentaculum tali, medially?

157. Explain why the heads of the 2nd, 3rd and 4th metatarsals are more difficult to palpate from below.

158. Describe the deformity in the condition of 'hammer toes'. (fr)

159. Describe the head of the proximal phalanx.

160. On inversion and eversion, what movement occurs at the tubercle of the navicula?

Please complete the labels below.

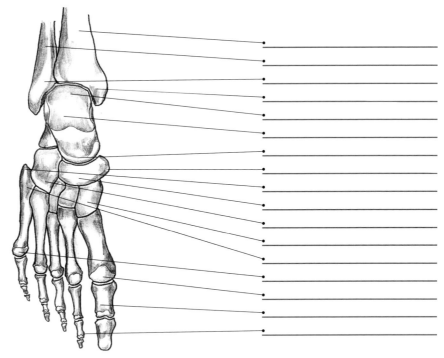

Fig. 2.7 (b) Bones of the right foot (dorsal aspect)

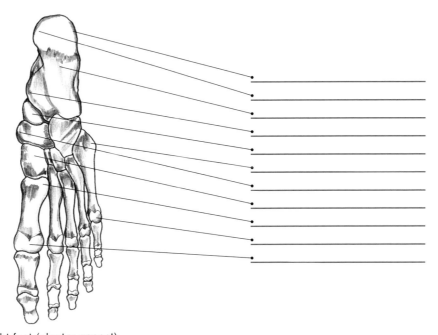

Fig. 2.8 (b) Bones of the right foot (plantar aspect)

Chapter 3
Joints

Contents

The lumbar spine   58
The pelvis   62
The pubic symphysis   62
The sacroiliac joint   64
The hip joint   66
The knee joint   68
The tibiofibular union   72
    The superior tibiofibular joint   72
    The inferior tibiofibular joint   73
The ankle joint   74
The foot   78
    The talocalcaneal (subtalar) joint   78
    The talocalcaneonavicular joint   82
    The calcaneocuboid joint   84
    The cuboideonavicular joint   85
    The midtarsal joint   85
    The cuneonavicular and intercuneiform joints   86
    The tarsometatarsal joints   87
    The intermetatarsal joints   88
    The metatarsophalangeal joints   90
    The interphalangeal joints   92
Self-assessment questions   94

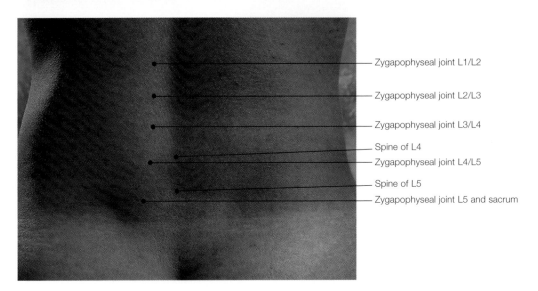

Zygapophyseal joint L1/L2

Zygapophyseal joint L2/L3

Zygapophyseal joint L3/L4

Spine of L4

Zygapophyseal joint L4/L5

Spine of L5

Zygapophyseal joint L5 and sacrum

Fig. 3.1 (a)
The zygapophyseal joints of lumbar spine (posterior view)

THE LUMBAR SPINE [Fig. 3.1]

The **zygapophyseal joints** are the most superficial in the lumbar region. They are nevertheless covered by thick, strong muscle, making the task of palpation extremely difficult. With the fingers pressed between the sides of the **vertebral spines** and the parallel-running column of muscle (sacrospinalis), the sides of the spines and in some subjects the **laminae** of each vertebra may be palpated. Each is a little higher than its corresponding spine, being almost totally hidden by the thick muscle layer.

Deep pressure through the muscle, using the tips of the thumbs, applies pressure to the posterior aspect of the zygapophyseal joints, which lie 1 cm lateral and slightly lower than the vertebral spine. With great care and precision this pressure can be targeted onto the upper articular pillar of the vertebra below by moving lateral to the joint, or onto the lower articular pillar of the vertebra above by moving just medial to the joint. The lower facets of the vertebrae are convex anteriorly and fit snugly into the concave anterior edge of the upper facets of the vertebra below. Thus, anterior pressure on the lower vertebra causes its articular facet to glide forwards, slightly parting its anterior segments, whereas pressure on the upper vertebra pushes the lower facet into the socket, preventing any further movement (Fig. 3.1d,e).

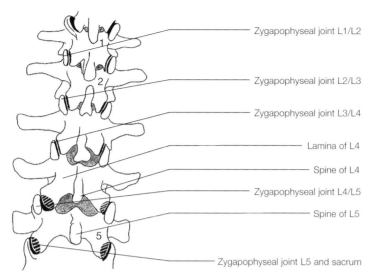

Fig. 3.1 (b)
The zygapophyseal joints of lumbar spine (posterior view)

Zygapophyseal joint L1/L2

Zygapophyseal joint L2/L3

Zygapophyseal joint L3/L4

Lamina of L4

Spine of L4

Zygapophyseal joint L4/L5

Spine of L5

Zygapophyseal joint L5 and sacrum

Accessory movements

Distraction (traction) of the joints of the lumbar spine is the only true accessory movement possible. All other movements of gliding, gapping and compression of the zygapophyseal joints, together with twisting and compression of the intervertebral discs, occur in the area during normal lumbar activities.

Traction can be applied to this area in many ways, either manually or mechanically. The lumbar column, however, can be placed in many different positions to achieve the therapeutic result required.

Extension of the lumbar spine tends to create a 'close-packed' position for the individual joints, as the articular surfaces come into full contact and ligaments become taut. This, therefore, is not a desirable position in which to achieve traction. All other positions towards flexion allow space for the joint surfaces to part or glide; however, in full flexion the ligaments again become taut, preventing the required movements. Traction in full flexion is almost impossible to apply. The optimum position in which to apply traction is midway between extension and flexion.

Simple traction can be applied to the lumbar spine by applying a distraction force to either the pelvis or the lower limbs, with the subject lying either supine or prone. It is preferable to place a pillow under the abdomen in the latter position to prevent extension. Manual traction can also be applied with the subject sitting or standing, by raising the upper trunk and allowing the pelvis and lower limbs to act as the traction force.

Mechanical traction can be applied in many positions of the lumbar spine, avoiding full extension and full flexion for the same reasons as outlined above. It may be applied continuously or intermittently over a set period of time. These therapeutic traction techniques are complex and need skill and knowledge of techniques and precautions. For further study, reference should be made to literature dedicated to this subject.

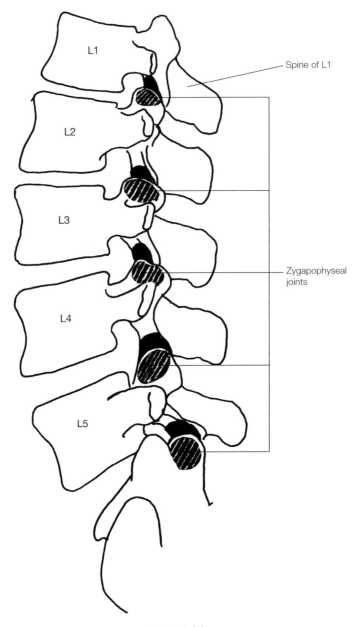

Fig. 3.1 (c)
The zygapophyseal joints of the lumbar spine (lateral aspect from left)

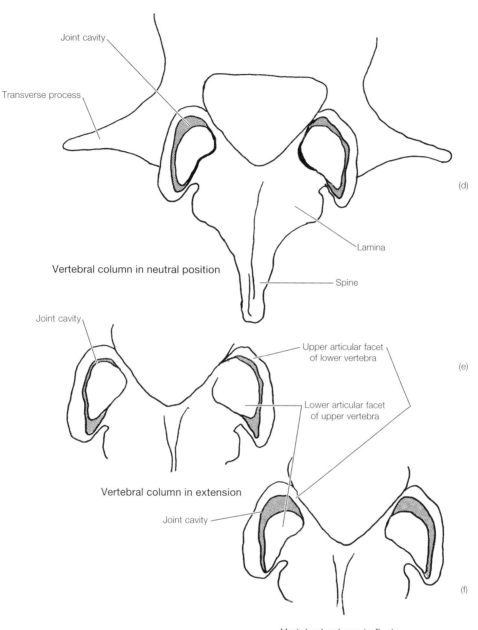

Joint cavity

Transverse process

Lamina

Spine

Vertebral column in neutral position

(d)

Joint cavity

Upper articular facet
of lower vertebra

(e)

Lower articular facet
of upper vertebra

Vertebral column in extension

Joint cavity

(f)

Vertebral column in flexion

Fig. 3.1 (d)–(f)
The zygapophyseal joints of lumbar section of vertebral column (viewed from above)

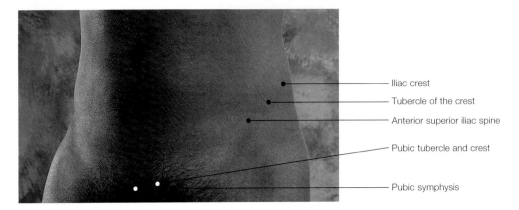

Iliac crest

Tubercle of the crest

Anterior superior iliac spine

Pubic tubercle and crest

Pubic symphysis

Fig. 3.2 (a)
The pelvis (anterior view)

THE PELVIS [Fig. 3.2]

Posteriorly, the **sacrum** articulates on either side with the **ilium** (innominate) bone at the **sacroiliac joints**. Anteriorly, the two pubic bodies articulate with each other at the pubic symphysis. The former is a very stable plane synovial joint supported by powerful interosseous and accessory ligaments. The latter is also stable, but is a secondary cartilaginous joint containing a modified disc of fibrocartilage. The sacroiliac joints allow a small degree of rotation of the sacrum, with respect to the innominate bones, about an axis through its interosseous ligament. Movement is more noticeable in young females, particularly during pregnancy and childbirth, reducing considerably after the third decade. In males, movement is negligible and virtually nil after the second decade.

The pubic symphysis allows a slight rocking and twisting to occur, which accompanies any movements which may occur at the sacroiliac joints.

THE PUBIC SYMPHYSIS

This joint is situated centrally at the lower aspect of the abdomen between the two **pubic bones** and just above the external genitalia. Locate the **pubic tubercles** on the upper border of the body of the pubis, either

side of the midline. Between the two is a depressed line which can be traced downwards for about 2.5 cm. This indicates the anterior marking of the **pubic symphysis**, being the medial surfaces of the pubic bones separated only by the intervening interarticular disc.

Accessory movements

The slight twisting and gapping that occurs at this joint is due to stresses on the pelvis and sacrum which occur during movements at the sacroiliac and hip joint. With the subject lying supine, a slight gliding movement can be produced between the two bones by applying pressure to the anterior surface of the pubic body on one side only.

With the subject lying on the side, a downward compression force applied to the upper part of the ilium increases compression at the pubic symphysis, while also stressing the posterior sacroiliac ligament. With the subject supine, the two ilia can be stressed laterally by a downward and lateral pressure being applied to the two **iliac crests**. This produces a distraction force to the pubic symphysis and, in addition, an anterior gapping and stress on the anterior ligament of the **sacroiliac joint**.

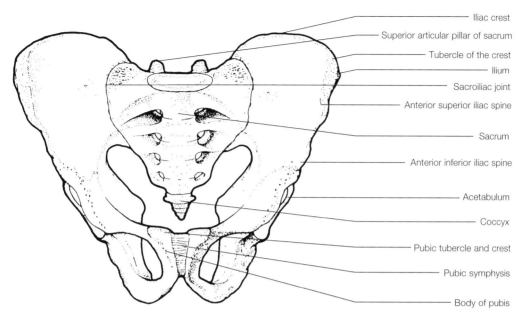

Iliac crest
Superior articular pillar of sacrum
Tubercle of the crest
Ilium
Sacroiliac joint
Anterior superior iliac spine
Sacrum
Anterior inferior iliac spine
Acetabulum
Coccyx
Pubic tubercle and crest
Pubic symphysis
Body of pubis

Fig. 3.2 (b)
The pelvis (anterior view)

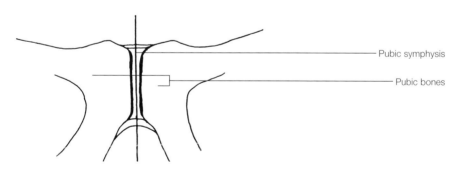

Pubic symphysis
Pubic bones

Fig. 3.2 (c)
The pelvis (anterior view)

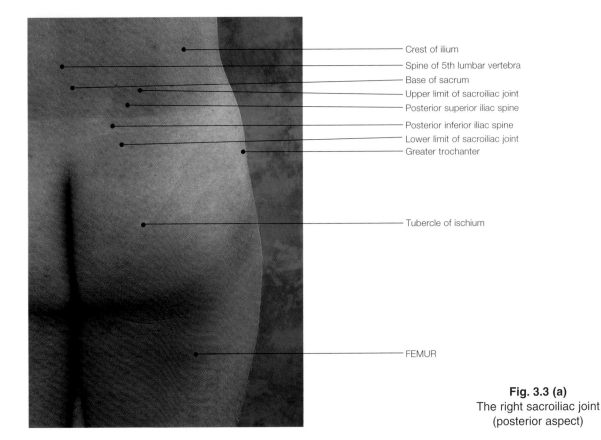

Crest of ilium
Spine of 5th lumbar vertebra
Base of sacrum
Upper limit of sacroiliac joint
Posterior superior iliac spine
Posterior inferior iliac spine
Lower limit of sacroiliac joint
Greater trochanter

Tubercle of ischium

FEMUR

Fig. 3.3 (a)
The right sacroiliac joint
(posterior aspect)

THE SACROILIAC JOINT

Structure

This joint is situated deeply in the back of the pelvis and is formed by the auricular surface on the lateral side of the sacrum and the sacropelvic surface of the hip bone. It is a synovial joint surrounded by a capsule and lined with synovial membrane. The capsule is supported by anterior, posterior and interosseous ligaments and the joint is further supported by two accessory ligaments, the sacrotuberous and the sacrospinous.

Palpation and surface marking

This joint is set deeply at the back of the pelvis and is thus difficult to palpate. Nevertheless, certain landmarks can be identified, giving an accurate indication of its position (Fig. 3.3). With the subject lying prone and the abdomen resting on a pillow, identify the **posterior superior iliac spine**. The sacroiliac joint lies 1 cm lateral and 1 cm anterior to this spine, on an oblique line extending above and below a further 2 cm.. Find the **posterior superior** and **inferior iliac**

spines (Fig. 3.3b). The line of the joint can be marked by an oblique line passing downwards and medially at an angle of approximately 25° from a point 5 cm lateral to the **spine of the fifth lumbar vertebra** to a point just lateral to the posterior inferior iliac spine. It is impossible to actually palpate this joint. The joint is, however, in a plane running forwards and laterally under the posterior part of the ilium, reaching as far forward as the apex of the greater sciatic notch (Fig. 3.4b).

Accessory movements

There is much controversy concerning the movements that may occur at this joint. The fact that it is a synovial joint with plane, although irregular, articular surfaces suggests that it is designed for movement. However, the irregularity of the articular surface, together with the presence of extremely strong, short interosseous ligaments, means that in reality little

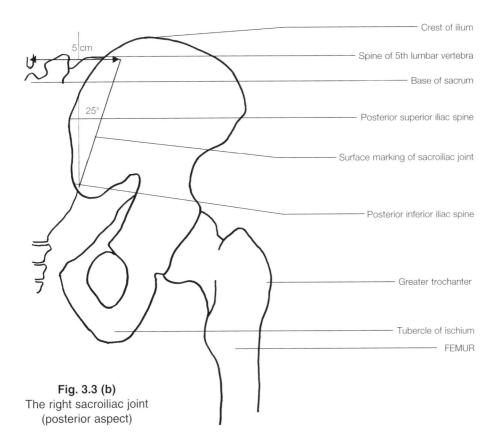

5 cm

25°

Crest of ilium

Spine of 5th lumbar vertebra

Base of sacrum

Posterior superior iliac spine

Surface marking of sacroiliac joint

Posterior inferior iliac spine

Greater trochanter

Tubercle of ischium

FEMUR

Fig. 3.3 (b)
The right sacroiliac joint
(posterior aspect)

movement is possible. In the young female, move-ment is often considerable, whereas in the elderly male, little or no movement is possible. The two joints on either side of the **sacrum** and the symphysis pubis anteriorly allow slight rotation and gapping move-ments to occur, which reduce the stresses imparted on the pelvis from the trunk and lower limbs.

Slight rotation of the sacrum forwards and back-wards around a frontal axis running through its inter-osseous ligament may be regarded as normal physio-logical movement. It can, however, be aided by press-ure placed alternately on the upper and lower aspects of its posterior surface, with the subject in prone lying, thereby rocking the sacrum between the ilia. The opposite movement can be produced by placing one hand on the base of the sacrum and the other on the ischial tuberosity. The pressure applied to these two areas must be downwards and towards each other, in the same direction as the movement of each compon-ent. It is a difficult movement to obtain, and some skill and practice is necessary before it can be achieved.

Rotation of the ilium can be enhanced by using the **femur** as a lever and localizing the movement of the joint with the other hand. With the subject lying on one side, stand behind the hip region and take the upper femur into extension; the other hand should be placed on the posterior aspect of the **iliac crest**. Considerable fixation of the rest of the pelvis can be achieved if the subject holds the alternate knee up to the chest. Flexion of the femur on the pelvis produces a backward rotation of the ilium on the sacrum, which can be enhanced by pressure applied from the front on the anterior superior iliac spine, and fixation by the subject extending the alternate lower limb. With the subject supine, slight gapping of the posterior part of the sacroiliac joint can be achieved by rotating the pelvis and flexed lower limb to the side and apply-ing a downward and inward pressure on the femur, towards the hip. During these movements, associated gapping and twisting occur at the pubic symphysis. For additional information consult the manipulation literature.

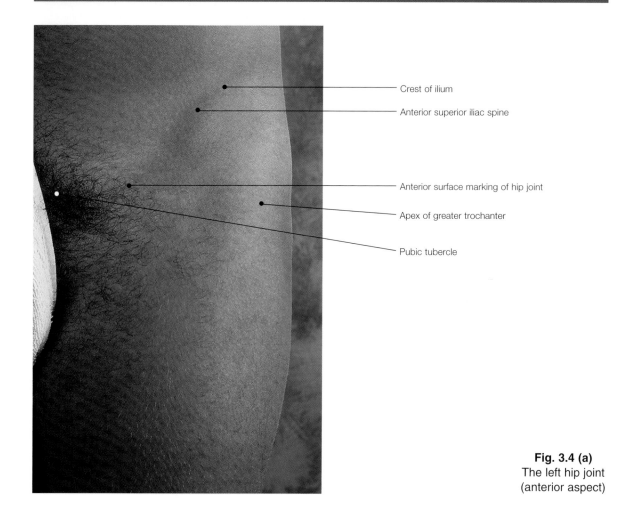

Crest of ilium

Anterior superior iliac spine

Anterior surface marking of hip joint

Apex of greater trochanter

Pubic tubercle

Fig. 3.4 (a)
The left hip joint
(anterior aspect)

THE HIP JOINT [Fig. 3.4]

This is a large synovial ball-and-socket joint between the head of the femur and the acetabulum of the hip bone. It lies on the anterolateral aspect of the pelvis and affords a considerable amount of mobility to the lower limb. It is surrounded by a capsule which encloses a large part of the femoral neck, both lined with synovial membrane. The capsule is supported, externally, by the very powerful iliofemoral, ischio-femoral and pubofemoral ligaments. In addition further support is afforded internally by the ligament of the head deep inside the joint and the acetabular labrum, which attaches to the rim of the acetabulum and transverse ligament, thus surrounding the head.

Surface marking

The joint lies in the groin some 1.5 cm below the mid-point of the inguinal ligament, i.e. halfway between the **anterior superior iliac spine** and the **pubic tubercle** (see pages 20–21). The acetabulum extends 4 cm vertically below this point deep to the head of the femur. Midway between the upper and lower limits, i.e. at the midpoint of the joint, the acetabulum extends 2 cm either side of this vertical line (Fig. 3.4).

An alternative method of establishing the centre of the hip joint can be by tracing a line horizontally and medially from the upper border of the **greater trochanter** to a point below the midpoint of the inguinal ligament. When viewed posteriorly, the hip joint centre lies 5 cm above and 3 cm lateral to the ischial tuberosity.

Palpation

Palpation of the joint from any aspect is, however, virtually impossible as it is covered by thick muscle

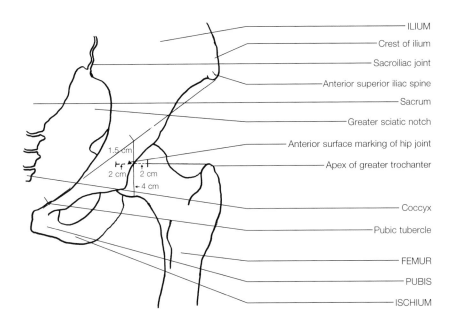

ILIUM
Crest of ilium
Sacroiliac joint
Anterior superior iliac spine
Sacrum
Greater sciatic notch
Anterior surface marking of hip joint
Apex of greater trochanter
Coccyx
Pubic tubercle
FEMUR
PUBIS
ISCHIUM

1.5 cm
2 cm   2 cm
4 cm

Fig. 3.4 (b)
The left hip joint
(anterior aspect)

crossing the joint, particularly posteriorly and later-ally. Only if the hip is fully extended can movement be detected and then only anteriorly. If the fingers are placed on the anterior surface marking of the joint, with the subject standing, and the limb is then taken into approximately 15° of extension, the head of the femur can be palpated projecting forwards under the anterior covering of muscles (iliopsoas and pectineus).

Accessory movements

There is very little accessory movement at this joint. With the subject lying supine and the hip flexed approximately 30°, slight parting of the articular surfaces is possible. This is produced by applying strong traction to the femur.

Movements of flexion, extension and rotation of the hip, however, with the hands carefully controlling

the movement from the lower end of the femur, can be a source of important information for the palpator. Quality and range of movement can be assessed and areas of 'grinding' and limitation can be located. Linked with the patient's symptoms and reactions, a much clearer picture of the problems involved can be visualized.

Combining the three components of movement, i.e. flexion/extension, abduction/adduction and medial/lateral rotation, can test the joint movement and funct-ion to extremes. Testing in these confined movements is often referred to as the 'quadrants' and for further information concerning these manoeuvres the manip-ulation and mobilization literature should be consulted (Maitland 1991). Fixation of proximal and distal joints in testing of the hip joint is essential, as compensatory movement is common in this area and can lead to incorrect diagnosis.

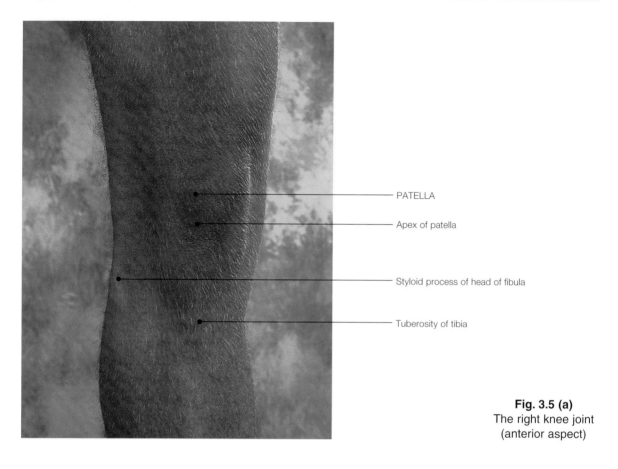

PATELLA

Apex of patella

Styloid process of head of fibula

Tuberosity of tibia

Fig. 3.5 (a)
The right knee joint
(anterior aspect)

THE KNEE JOINT [Fig. 3.5]

The knee joint is a synovial composite joint comprising the bicondylar section between the condyles of **femur** and **tibia** and the plane joint between the **patella** and the patellar surface of the femur. The joint functions as a modified hinge, with the main movements being flexion and extension. Rotation can be produced in the semiflexed position and in the final few degrees of full extension.

It is the largest joint in the human body and perhaps the most complex (see *Anatomy and Human Movement*, Palastanga, Field and Soames 2002).

The articular surfaces are covered with articular cartilage, but are not congruent. Those on the femur cover the superior, posterior, inferior and anterior surfaces of the large condyles, coming together anteriorly to form a triangular surface which is narrow at the top and is called the patellar surface. The articular surfaces of the tibia only cover the central section of the upper surface; its outer sections are covered by two crescentic-shaped menisci.

The joint is supported on its posterior, lateral and medial side by a fibrous capsule. Anteriorly the capsule is formed by the lower section of the quadriceps femoris, the patella and the ligamentum patellae. The joint is lined by an extensive and complex synovial membrane and is supported by numerous ligaments, including the oblique popliteal, the tibial collateral, the fibula collateral externally and the anterior and posterior cruciate ligaments internally. It also relies heavily on the powerful surrounding muscles for its stability.

Anterior to the condylar section is the patellofemoral joint between the posterior surface of the patella and the patellar surface of the femur. This is a synovial plane joint, separate from the knee although it shares the same joint space and synovial membrane.

The knee joint appears at first sight to be a very unstable joint with the two rounded condyles of the femur sitting on top of the two flattened surfaces of the tibia. This, however, is not so. This joint rarely dislocates and even then only under extreme force, such as a car or aeroplane crash. It is, however, subject to many stresses and strains, particularly in sport.

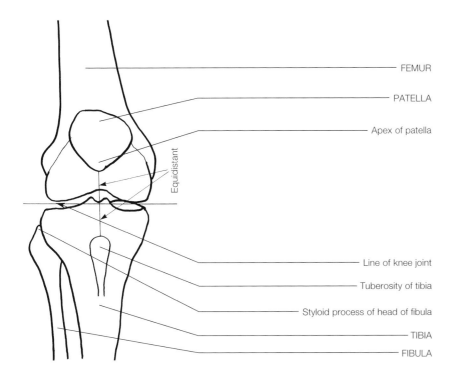

FEMUR

PATELLA

Apex of patella

Equidistant

Line of knee joint

Tuberosity of tibia

Styloid process of head of fibula

TIBIA

FIBULA

Fig. 3.5 (b)
The right knee joint
(anterior aspect)

Surface marking

The joint lies on a line which bisects the ligamentum patellae horizontally (Fig. 3.5b,d), **halfway between the lower tip of the patella and the tibial tuberosity**. An alternative method of marking the joint is by drawing a line horizontally 1 cm above the tip of the styloid process of the fibula.

Palpation

With the fingers either side of the ligamentum patellae, two triangular depressions can be felt. These are bounded by the tibia below, the femur above and the ligamentum patellae centrally. At the apex of the depression, running horizontally, is the knee joint space; your fingers are now resting against the anterior aspect of the medial and lateral menisci. These can be observed moving forwards during rotation at the joint, the lateral meniscus on lateral rotation and the medial on medial rotation. Tracing the joint posteriorly, the space becomes narrower until just behind the midpoint it becomes hidden by the medial collateral ligament medially and the lateral part of the joint capsule laterally. Posteriorly the joint is impossible to palpate due to the presence of muscle, tendon and fascial coverings, although the joint can be represented by a horizontal line drawn across the back of the popliteal fossa 1 cm above the tip of the styloid process of the head of the fibula (Fig. 3.5f).

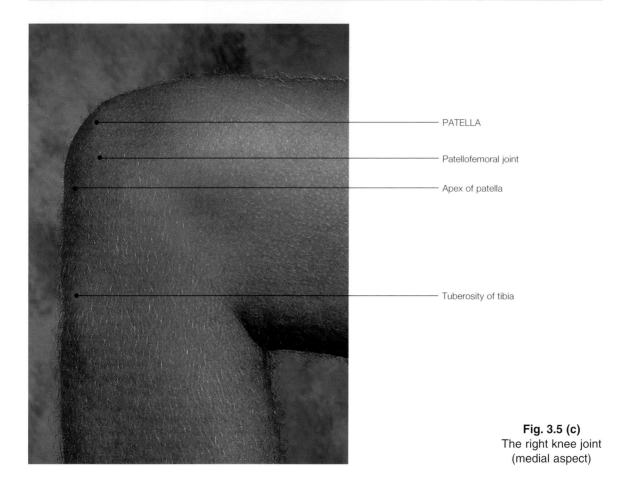

PATELLA

Patellofemoral joint

Apex of patella

Tuberosity of tibia

Fig. 3.5 (c)
The right knee joint
(medial aspect)

Accessory movements

The knee joint becomes 'close packed' on full extension; therefore, accessory movements should only be performed avoiding the extreme of extension. With the subject lying supine, the knee flexed to 90° and the foot firmly fixed on the supporting surface (often achieved by the investigator sitting on the foot), the tibial condyles can be drawn forwards (anterior draw test), and pushed backwards, producing a gliding of the tibial condyles against the femoral condyles. There should be only a slight movement in either direction, forward movement of the tibia being limited by the anterior cruciate ligament and posterior movement being limited by the posterior cruciate ligament.

With the subject again lying supine with the knee flexed 15°, stabilize the under-surface of the thigh with one hand and grasp the lower end of the leg just above the ankle with the other. A side-to-side movement can be produced. Distraction of the joint can also be achieved by pulling on the leg in the mid-position, with the subject seated on a high plinth with the foot clear of the floor.

The **patellofemoral joint** lies deep to the **patella**, between it and the patellar surface of the femur, 1 cm deep to its anterior surface (Fig. 3.5c,d), sharing the same joint space as the bicondylar articulation. It is easily marked by tracing around the perimeter of bone. When the knee is in an extended and relaxed position, the patella can be moved from side to side across the patellar surface of the femur, resulting in a knocking effect. It can also be moved up and down as a gliding movement along the vertical groove of the femoral surface.

With the patella moved laterally, the medial edge of the patellar surface of the femur can be palpated, marked by a sharp ridge. In this position, the under-surface of the lateral edge of the patella can also be palpated. Conversely, if the patella is moved medially, the lateral edge of the patellar surface of the femur and the medial under-surface of the patella also become palpable.

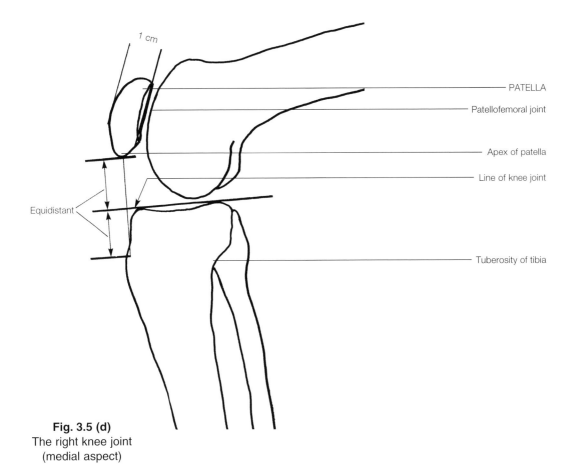

Fig. 3.5 (d)
The right knee joint
  (medial aspect)

Functional anatomy

Little stress is applied to the structural components of the knee joint, on which it relies for its stability during normal activities, such as walking, running, jumping, swimming, etc. However, enormous tension is applied to these components during sporting activities where the lower limbs are used for varied directional propulsion and kicking. Lateral or medial forces applied to the knee, particularly when the knee is in its extended 'close-packed' position may cause strains, partial tears or even complete ruptures to medial or lateral ligaments. Violent over-extension of the knee may rupture the anterior cruciate ligament, and the posterior cruciate ligament may rupture when enormous force is applied to the anterior aspect of the proximal end of the tibia. When the knee is over-rotated in a flexed position the menisci, especially the medial, sometimes get trapped between the rolling condyle of the femur on the tibia, producing a tear in the meniscus.

In addition to all the ligamentous problems, the very powerful muscle surrounding the joint, on which stability is also dependent, may be partially torn or even completely ruptured. On a violent extension force such as kicking a stationary object, or falling from a height on to the feet, the quadriceps femoris tendon may rupture causing complete dysfunction of the joint.

When one considers all the fractures that may occur through direct or indirect violence to the bones of the joint and the degeneration due to age and all the stresses applied by virtually the whole body weight being transferred through the joint during movement, it is hardly surprising that the knee joints are a source of much pain and suffering, for many, in their senior years.

(For detailed study of structure, stability, function, dysfunction, remedies, etc., see *Anatomy and Human Movement*, Palastanga, Field and Soames 2002.)

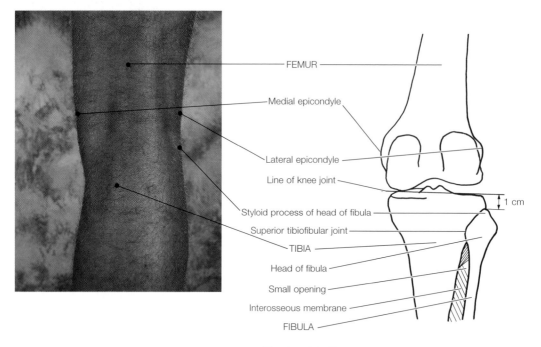

Fig. 3.5 (e), (f)
The right knee joint (posterior aspect)

THE TIBIOFIBULAR UNION

The **tibia** and **fibula** are joined together by two joints, the **superior tibiofibular joint** and the **inferior tibiofibular joint**, and an **interosseous membrane**. They unite the bones so tightly that very little movement occurs between the two. The interosseous membrane is composed of strong fibrous tissue with its fibres passing downwards and laterally. There is a **small opening** above (see Fig. 3.5f), with an additional group of fibres passing in the opposite direction just below the superior tibiofibular joint.

The superior tibiofibular joint

This is a synovial joint, with its surfaces covered with articular cartilage and it is surrounded by a capsule lined with synovial membrane. The capsule is supported by the anterior and posterior tibiofibular ligaments.

Surface marking

This joint can be represented, both anteriorly and posteriorly, by a line 1.5 cm in length running downwards and slightly medially just medial to the head of the fibula (Fig. 3.6a,b).

Palpation

With the model in supine lying and the knee straight, stand on the right side just below the level of the knee. Place the index finger of your left hand on the styloid process of the head of the fibula. From that point your thumb can trace downwards and medially along the anterior aspect of the joint. Your middle finger is just behind the joint, and similarly to the thumb, can trace downwards and medially along the posterior joint line. This is a little more difficult to palpate as it is covered by the lateral head of gastrocnemius.

Accessory movements

Although the head of the fibula can be felt gliding up and down during dorsiflexion and plantar flexion of the ankle joint, accessory movement between the two bones is virtually impossible. With the subject lying supine and the ankle joint plantar flexed, direct pressure, applied by the thumb, on the head of the fibula can produce a slight backward gliding. Forward gliding can be achieved using the same technique but with the subject lying prone. Extreme care must be taken, when performing this procedure, to avoid the common peroneal nerve as it winds around the neck of the fibula.

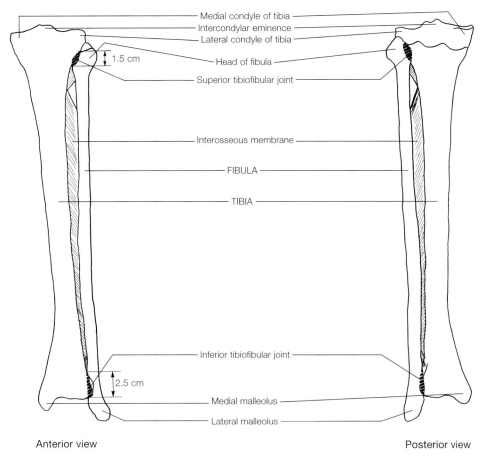

Fig. 3.6 (a), (b)
The superior and inferior tibiofibular joints and union of the left side

The inferior tibiofibular joint

This joint is a fibrous syndesmosis [*syndesmos* (Gk) = a band] between the lower lateral rough triangular surface on the tibia and a similar surface on the lower medial side of the fibula. The surfaces are bound together by a very strong interosseous ligament which is a continuation downwards of the interosseous membrane. The joint is further supported by an anterior, posterior and transverse tibiofibular ligament, the latter forming part of the socket of the ankle joint.

Surface marking

This joint can be represented by a vertical line 2.5 cm long running superiorly from the line of the ankle joint (see page 74) on the medial side of the **lateral malleolus**.

Palpation

Again it is difficult to palpate, except for its upper edge, as it is mostly covered by the superior extensor retinaculum and extensor digitorum longus tendons. Posteriorly, little can be palpated owing to the presence of the tendocalcaneus.

Accessory movements

Accessory movement of the inferior tibiofibular joint is not possible, except when diastasis (a parting of the inferior tibiofibular joint) has occurred. It is unwise to increase the unwanted movement in this injury, as this leads to even further instability of the ankle joint.

The fibrous interosseous ligament between the two bones holds the two bones together and is referred to by some as a fibrous syndesmosis.

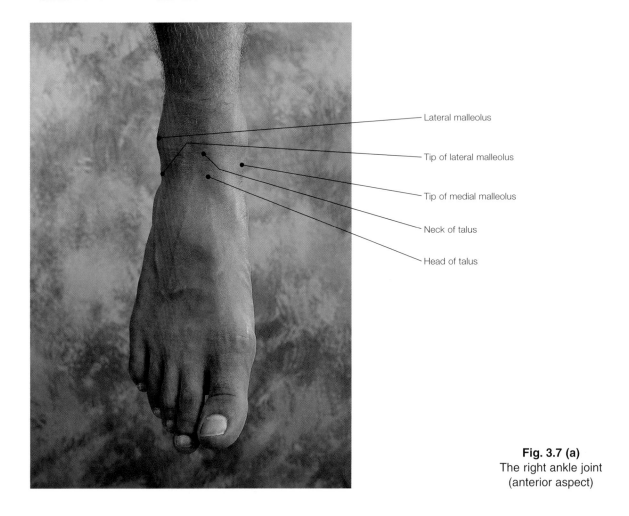

Lateral malleolus

Tip of lateral malleolus

Tip of medial malleolus

Neck of talus

Head of talus

Fig. 3.7 (a)
The right ankle joint
(anterior aspect)

THE ANKLE JOINT [Fig. 3.7]

The ankle joint is a synovial hinge joint involving the distal ends of the **tibia** and **fibula** proximally and the **body of the talus** distally. The weight-bearing surfaces are the trochlear surfaces of the tibia and talus. The stabilizing surfaces are those of the **medial** and **lateral malleoli**, which grip the body of the talus. The articular surfaces are composed of, above, the inferior surface of the tibia, the medial surface of the lateral malleolus and lateral surface of the medial malleolus, and, below, the superior, lateral and upper part of the medial surface of the talus. The surfaces are covered with articular cartilage. The joint is surrounded by a capsule lined with synovial membrane and is supported by very powerful lateral and medial (deltoid) ligaments. These two ligaments are delta-shaped, being narrower above and broader below. Above they are attached to the anterior and posterior borders, tip and

fossae of each malleolus. Below, the medial attaches to the navicular, calcaneonavicular 'spring' ligament, sustentaculum tali and medial tubercle of talus, with a deep section attaching to the medial surface of the talus. The lateral has three portions, the anterior and posterior attaching to the talus and the middle portion to the calcaneus. The transverse tibiofibular ligament which passes across the posterior of the ankle joint, forming part of its socket, attaches to both malleoli and the lower border of the tibia.

A horizontal line drawn across the anterior surface of the ankle 2 cm above the tip of the medial and 3 cm above that of the lateral malleolus marks the superior limit of the joint. It is continued down the medial side of the lateral malleolus and the lateral side of the medial malleolus to their tips which completes the joint line (Fig. 3.7b,d,f).

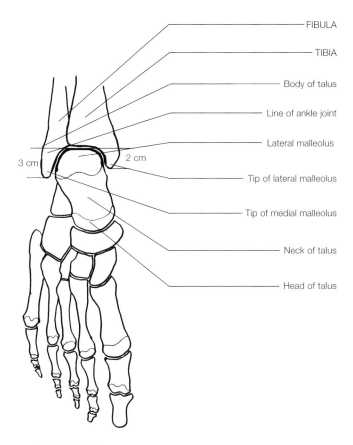

FIBULA

TIBIA

Body of talus

Line of ankle joint

Lateral malleolus

3 cm   2 cm

Tip of lateral malleolus

Tip of medial malleolus

Neck of talus

Head of talus

Fig. 3.7 (b)
The right ankle joint
(anterior aspect)

Palpation

Careful palpation between the extensor tendons in the region of the horizontal part of the joint line reveals the lower border of the tibia. Medially the joint line can be traced onto the anterior border of the medial malleolus and down to the tip. It can be traced up the posterior border of the medial malleolus, above the malleolar fossa where the joint line is hidden by tissue which lies between the tendocalcaneus and the joint. Laterally the joint line can be palpated between the talus and lateral malleolus anteriorly, and can be traced down to the tip of the malleolus. As on the medial side, its posterior border can be traced upwards above the malleolar fossa until it too is lost under similar fascia. With the ankle plantarflexed, the body of the talus, i.e. its upper, lateral and medial surfaces, can be felt gliding forwards (Fig. 3.7c,d). Posteriorly the joint is hidden by tendons and fascia.

Accessory movements

The ankle joint allows the movements of dorsiflexion and plantarflexion. Side-to-side movement is limited by the presence of the two malleoli, there being no movement possible when the joint is dorsiflexed and 'close packed' as the body is gripped between the two malleoli. However, when the joint is plantarflexed, by gripping the foot with one hand and stabilizing the leg with the other, the narrower part of the body of the talus can be moved from side to side, as well as forwards and backwards.

Commonly the lateral (and less frequently the medial) malleolus is fractured by a lateromedial or mediolateral force. Unless the malleolus is replaced exactly, the talus is able to move sideways and the joint becomes less stable. The same mechanical problem will occur if the two bones are parted at the inferior tibiofibular joint (diastasis – see page 73).

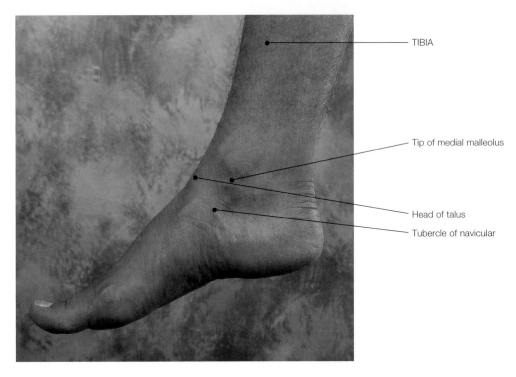

TIBIA

Tip of medial malleolus

Head of talus

Tubercle of navicular

Fig. 3.7 (c)
The right ankle joint (medial aspect)

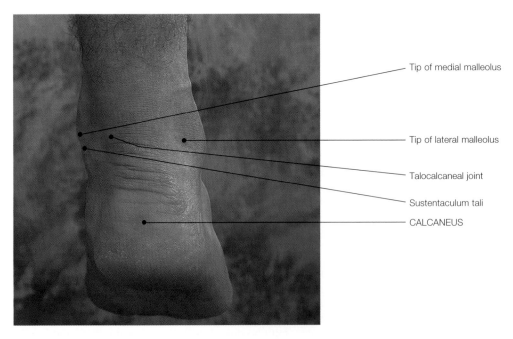

Tip of medial malleolus

Tip of lateral malleolus

Talocalcaneal joint

Sustentaculum tali

CALCANEUS

Fig. 3.7 (e)
The right ankle joint (posterior aspect)

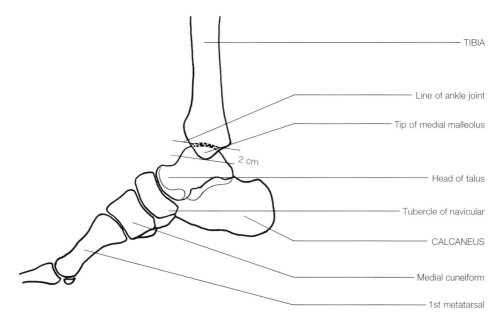

Fig. 3.7 (d)
The right ankle joint (medial aspect)

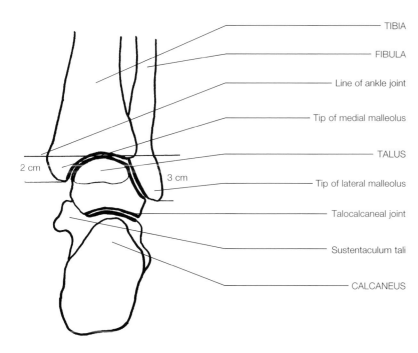

Fig. 3.7 (f)
The right ankle joint (posterior aspect)

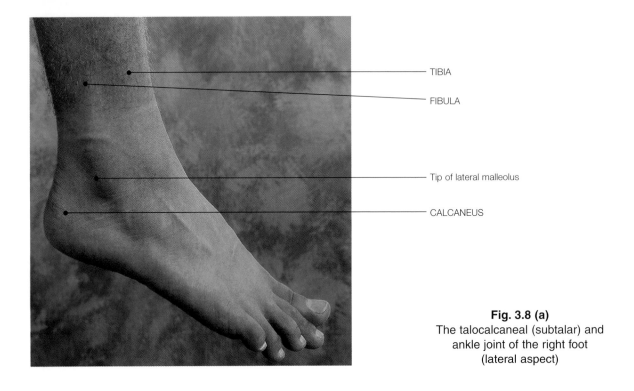

TIBIA

FIBULA

Tip of lateral malleolus

CALCANEUS

Fig. 3.8 (a)
The talocalcaneal (subtalar) and
ankle joint of the right foot
(lateral aspect)

THE FOOT

The joints of the foot are divided into those between the tarsal bones (the intertarsal joints) and the tarsal and metatarsal bones (the tarsometatarsal joints); those between the metatarsal bases (the intermetatarsal joints); those between the metatarsals and phalanges (the metatarsophalangeal joints); and those between the phalanges (the interphalangeal joints). Most of the joints are readily identifiable on the dorsum of the foot as they are only covered by thin fascia and the tendons of the long extensor muscles, whereas the plantar aspect of the foot is covered by numerous intrinsic muscles, in four layers, and very thick layers (up to 80) of plantar fascia.

The talocalcaneal (subtalar) joint [Fig. 3.8]

The **talocalcaneal** joint lies below the **talus** and is often referred to as the subtalar joint. The joint surf-

aces taking part in this joint are the inferior surface of the talus and the middle section of the superior surface of the calcaneus. Both surfaces are covered with articular cartilage and the joint is surrounded by a fibrous capsule lined with synovial membrane. The capsule is supported by medial, posterior, lateral and interosseous ligament. The interosseous ligament lies anterior to the joint and separates it from the talocalcaneonavicular joint. There is also a short ligament which joins the neck of the talus to the sustentaculum tali at the lateral end of the sinus tarsi.

Surface marking

The joint is marked by a line running horizontally 1 cm below the tip of the lateral malleolus on the lateral side to a point 1.5 cm below the tip of the medial malleolus on the medial side (Fig. 3.8b).

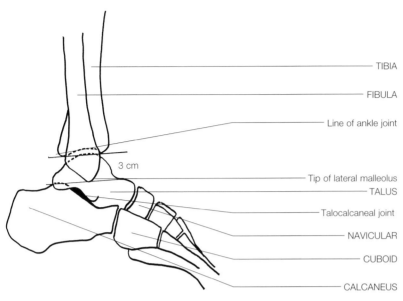

Fig. 3.8 (b)
The talocalcaneal (subtalar) and
ankle joint of the right foot
(lateral aspect)

Palpation

This is a very difficult joint to palpate due to the fact that the medial and lateral malleoli and the powerful ligaments tend to hide the joint. Find the tip of the lateral malleolus and move forward into the hollow. Below your finger you will feel the sharp edge of the upper border of the **calcaneus**. This is the anterior part of the lateral side of the joint.

On the medial side find the tip of the **medial malleolus**. Move down 2 cm and you will be able to palpate a horizontal ridge. This is the medial edge of the **sustentaculum tali** and its upper border is the lower boundary of the subtalar joint.

Accessory movement

With the model in supine lying, stand to the lateral side of the right foot (similar to the position adopted for accessory movements of the ankle joint). With your left hand grip the neck of the talus with your finger on the medial side and thumb laterally. With your right hand fit the model's heel into your palm with your fingers wrapping around the back of the calcaneus. The calcaneus can be rocked from side to side producing a slight gapping of the lateral and medial side of the joint alternately. The calcaneus can also be made to glide very slightly backwards and forwards.

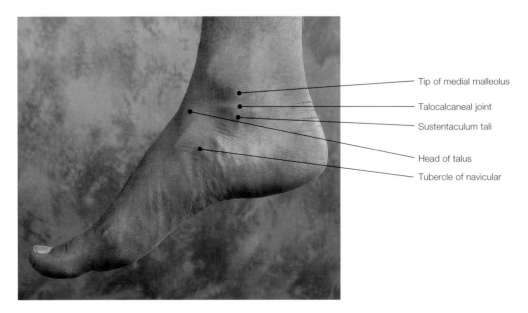

Fig. 3.8 (c)
The right talocalcaneal (subtalar) joint (medial aspect)

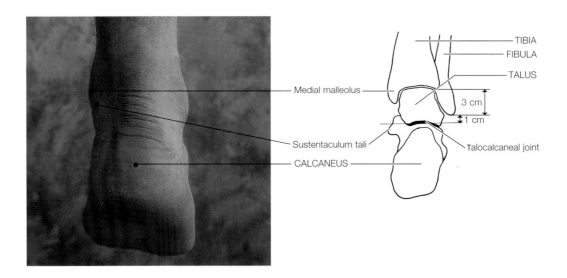

Fig. 3.8 (e), (f)
The talocalcaneal (subtalar) joint (posterior aspect)

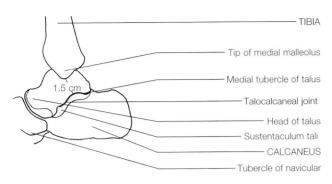

Fig. 3.8 (d)
The right talocalcaneal (subtalar) joint (medial aspect)

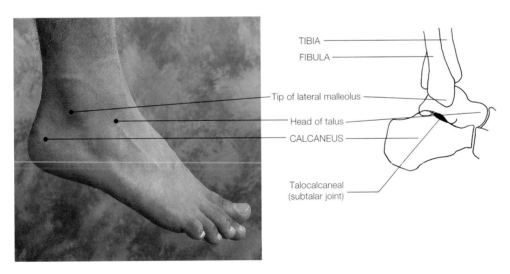

Fig. 3.8 (g), (h)
The talocalcaneal (subtalar) joint of the right foot (lateral aspect)

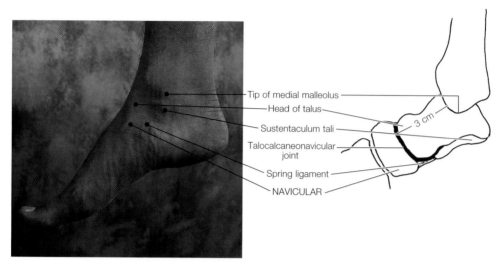

Tip of medial malleolus
Head of talus
Sustentaculum tali
Talocalcaneonavicular joint
Spring ligament
NAVICULAR

3 cm

Fig. 3.9 (a), (b)
The talocalcaneonavicular joint of right foot (medial aspect)

The talocalcaneonavicular joint
[Fig. 3.9a–d]

This is a synovial, modified ball-and-socket joint between the **head of the talus** and a socket comprising the posterior surface of **navicular**, the superior surface of the **sustentaculum tali** of the calcaneus and the 'spring' ligament which joins the two (Fig. 3.9). It is surrounded by a capsule lined with synovial membrane and is supported by the talonavicular ligament dorsally, the medial band of the bifurcate ('Y'-shaped) ligament laterally, the tibionavicular part of the deltoid ligament medially and posteroinferiorly, under the neck, by the anterior section of the interosseous ligament in the sinus tarsi. The plantar calcaneonavicular (spring) ligament is a fibroelastic ligament forming part of the socket and lies below the head of the talus, having articular cartilage on its superior surface.

Surface marking

The surface marking of the joint can be represented by a line, convex distally, drawn transversely across the medial half of the dorsum of the foot at the level of the tubercle of the navicular.

As with nearly all the joints in the foot, palpation and identification is only possible on the dorsum. The plantar aspect is hidden deep to many layers of the plantar fascia, many short but powerful muscles and strong, dense ligaments.

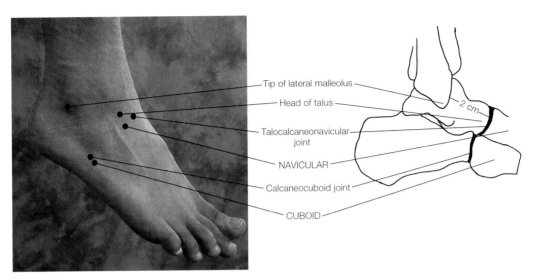

Fig. 3.9 (c), (d)
The talocalcaneonavicular and calcaneocuboid joints of right foot (lateral aspect)

Palpation

The tubercle of the navicular is situated 2.5 cm antero-inferior to the **tip of the medial malleolus** and is clearly palpable. As it projects slightly backwards, it is in line with the joint. The head of the talus can be traced down the proximal side of the tubercle to a small gap underneath, housing the 'spring' ligament. Posterior to the gap, the anterior section of the susten-taculum tali is palpable. If the foot is held in slight plantarflexion and the muscles relaxed, the joint can be traced across the dorsum of the foot almost to the midpoint where the head of the talus and the navic-ular dip towards the bifurcate ligament. The tendons of tibialis anterior and extensor hallucis longus may have to be moved to the side to follow the line clearly.

Accessory movements

Stand lateral to the foot. With your proximal hand, stabilize the talus from the medial side with your fingers on the plantar and thumb on the dorsal aspect. With your distal hand, grasp the forefoot as far back-wards as the navicular, again with your fingers on the plantar and thumb on the dorsal aspect. Slight up-and-down gliding can be obtained of the navicular on the head of the talus. Rotation of the forefoot on the head of the talus is also possible, but this is of course movement normally occurring during inversion and eversion.

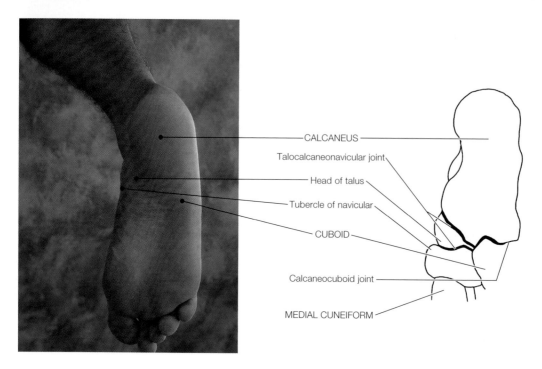

Fig. 3.9 (e), (f)
The talocalcaneonavicular and calcaneocuboid joint of right foot (plantar aspect)

The calcaneocuboid joint

This is a synovial, plane joint between the quadrilateral anterior surface of the calcaneus and the posterior surface of the cuboid. Both surfaces are covered with articular cartilage and the joint is surrounded by a capsule, lined with synovial membrane and supported by the lateral portion of the bifurcate ligament medially, by the dorsal calcaneocuboid ligament and by the plantar calcaneocuboid and long plantar ligaments.

Surface marking

The line of the joint is just proximal to the tubercle of the fifth metatarsal bone on the lateral and dorsal aspect of the base of the foot. It is slightly concave forwards.

Palpation

This joint is difficult to identify, although certain landmarks can be palpated. From the tip of the tubercle of the fifth metatarsal move dorsally 2 cm. Just proximal

to your finger you will feel the anterior border of the superior surface of the calcaneus. This is 2 cm anterior to the tip of the lateral malleolus. The border can be traced medially until it dips towards the bifurcate ligament, and laterally to the anterior border of the lateral surface almost down to the tubercle.

Accessory movement

This plane synovial joint allows slight upward movement during eversion and slight downward movement during inversion accompanying the rotation of the navicular on the **head of the talus**. This movement is physiological and its loss would severely interfere with the functional movement of the foot. With the model in supine lying, stand to the right of the right foot. Stabilize the talus and **calcaneus** by gripping below the two malleoli with the fingers on the inside. With the right hand, grasp the cuboid with the thumb on the dorsum and the index and middle fingers underneath. Now move the cuboid up and down. Note, only slight movement will be present.

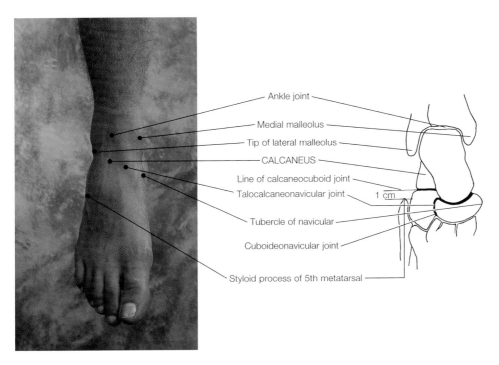

Fig. 3.9 (g), (h)
The midtarsal joint of the right foot (dorsal aspect)

The cuboideonavicular joint [Fig. 3.9h]

This joint between the navicular and the cuboid is normally a syndesmosis. The articular surfaces are joined entirely by a strong fibrous interosseous ligament and this is further supported by dorsal and plantar ligaments. Sometimes it is replaced by a small synovial joint which is surrounded by a capsule, lined by synovial membrane and supported by dorsal and plantar ligaments.

Surface marking

The joint is marked by a line 1 cm long running from back to front, 1 cm forward and 1 cm lateral to the lateral side of the head of the talus.

Palpation

The joint is impossible to palpate.

Accessory movements

As in all syndesmoses, there is usually a very minimal amount of movement, and as this restriction of movement is its function there is little point in trying to move the joint.

The midtarsal joint [Fig. 3.9g,h]

This is a composite articulation of the talocalcaneo-navicular joint medially and the **calcaneocuboid joint** laterally. The two proximal bones are firmly united by the interosseous ligament in the sinus tarsi and the two distal bones are firmly united by the cuboideo-navicular syndesmosis. The two joints are therefore considered to move as one unit, particularly in inversion and eversion of the foot.

Surface marking

The joint line can be marked across the dorsum of the foot by a line from just proximal to the tuberosity of the navicular medially to a point 1 cm proximal to the tip of the tubercle of the fifth metatarsal laterally (Fig. 3.9g,h).

Palpation

As in the separate joints above.

Accessory movements

As in the separate joints above.

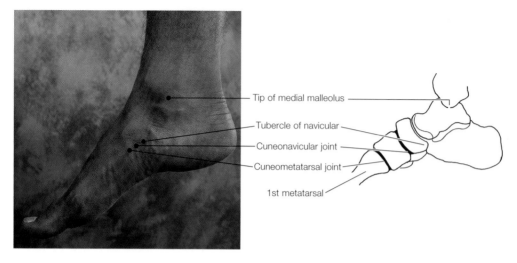

Fig. 3.9 (i), (j)
The cuneonavicular and cuneometatarsal joints of the right foot (medial aspect)

The cuneonavicular and intercuneiform joints [Figs 3.9i,j and 3.10c,d]

The three cuneiform bones articulate proximally with the distal surface of the navicular by plane synovial joints. They are surrounded by a common capsule which is lined by synovial membrane and is supported by relatively weak dorsal and stronger plantar ligaments. The cuneiform bones are also bound together distally by interosseous ligaments.

Palpation

The cuneonavicular joint can be palpated on its medial and dorsal aspects just distal to the navicular tuberosity and, with care, can be traced across the foot between the extensor tendons, being slightly concave proximally (Fig. 3.9i,j).

The joints between the cuneiforms themselves, and between the lateral cuneiform and the cuboid, are extremely difficult to palpate, although the joint lines can be determined by following proximally from the first, second and third metatarsal bones (Fig. 3.10a,b).

Accessory movements

The joints between the navicular and the cuneiforms, as well as those between the cuneiforms themselves, are all plane synovial joints but, as they also possess interosseous ligaments which bind the adjacent surfaces together, they possess very little movement. They can be moved passively by stabilizing the most proximal component with the fingers and thumb of one hand and gliding the distal component up and down with the other hand, the grip being similar to that used on the talocalcaneonavicular joint. Although only slight gliding is present at these joints, loss of this movement can lead to complete dysfunction of the foot.

The cuneocuboid joint is synovial but is also tightly bound together by an interosseous ligament, becoming, in part, a syndesmosis. Consequently, passive accessory movement between the two bones is virtually impossible.

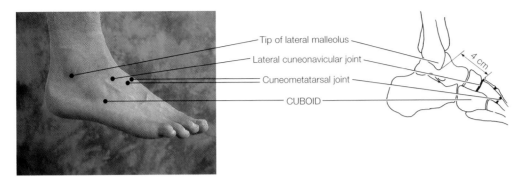

Fig. 3.10 (a), (b)
The cuneonavicular and cuneometatarsal joints of the right foot (lateral aspect)

The tarsometatarsal joints

The **tarsometatarsal joints** exist between the bases of the metatarsals and the cuneiform and cuboid bones. The first metatarsal articulates with the medial cuneiform bone, the second fits in between the medial and lateral cuneiforms with its base articulating with the middle, shorter, cuneiform, and the third metatarsal articulates with the lateral cuneiform. The fourth and fifth articulate with the cuboid. They are all plane synovial joints surrounded by a capsule which is lined with synovial membrane and supported by dorsal and plantar tarsometatarsal ligaments. There are also two or possibly three interosseous ligaments, two to the base of the second metatarsal as it fits into this mortice and the other between the lateral cuneiform to the fourth metatarsal.

Palpation and surface marking

The joint between the first metatarsal and the medial cuneiform can be palpated 2 cm distal to the navicular tuberosity. It can also be identified by following the first metatarsal proximally to where its base is marked by an expanded area. This line can be traced onto the dorsum of the foot, being crossed here by the tendon of extensor hallucis longus (Fig. 3.9i,j).

The joint between the second metatarsal and the middle cuneiform is extremely difficult to palpate as it is set more proximally between the medial and lateral cuneiforms. That between the third metatarsal and the lateral cuneiform, however, can be identified by following the line of the metatarsal to its base, which is slightly raised.

The same procedure will enable the joints between the fourth and fifth metatarsals and the cuboid to be identified. Its surface is marked by a line running laterally and proximally towards the tip of the tubercle on the fifth metatarsal (Figs 3.10a,b and 3.12a,b).

Accessory movements

With the model in supine lying, stand to the right of the right foot. With the cleft between your thumb and fingers of your left hand gripping the cuneiform bones and your right hand gripping the first metatarsal, movements up and down and even a little rotation can be obtained. There is a little movement obtained at these joints when the metatarsals are moved on each other (see The intermetatarsal joints, page 88).

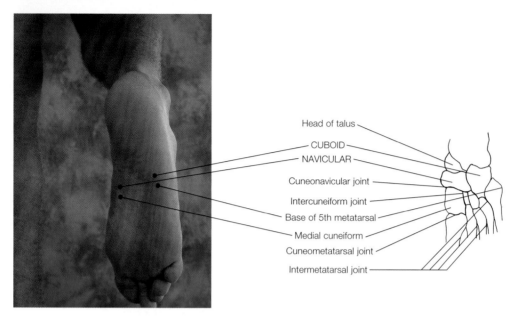

Fig. 3.10 (c), (d)
Joints of cuneiform bones and metatarsals of the right foot, plantar aspect (not palpable)

The intermetatarsal joints [Fig. 3.10c–f]

These are four small synovial joints between the adjacent sides of the bases of the second to fifth metatarsal. They are surrounded by a capsule lined with synovial membrane and their joint space is continuous with that of the tarsometatarsal joints. The capsule is supported by a dorsal and plantar ligament and an interosseous ligament at its distal end. The base of the first metatarsal is connected to the base of the second by an interosseous ligament only.

Surface marking

From a line drawn across the dorsum of the foot from the base of the first metatarsal to the tubercle on the base of the fifth, the joints pass distally for 0.5 cm in line with the spaces between the second to fifth metatarsal.

Palpation

If a finger is placed between the metatarsals on the dorsum of the foot and drawn proximally, the space between them gradually narrows, with the bones eventually coming into contact with each other. These small plane joints run anteroposteriorly for approximately 0.5 cm, as far proximally as the line drawn across the dorsum of the foot from the base of the first metatarsal and the tubercle on the lateral side of the base of the fifth. That between the second and third metatarsals is slightly smaller due to the arrangement of the cuneiforms (Fig. 3.10e,f).

The interosseous ligament between the first and second metatarsals can be marked in a similar fashion.

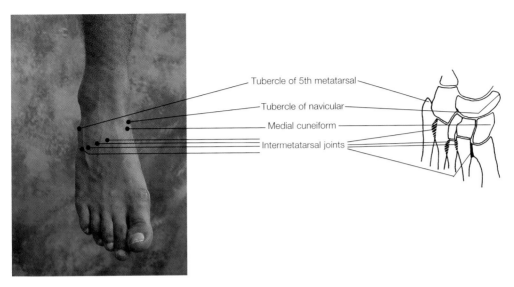

Fig. 3.10 (e), (f)
The intermetatarsal joints of the right foot (dorsal aspect)

Accessory movements

Movement between the metatarsal bases and either the **cuneiforms** or the **cuboid** is virtually non-existent. Only slight movements can be produced, even when the metatarsals are used as levers. Obviously this also results in a slight gliding movement at the intermetatarsal joints. With the subject lying supine, grip one metatarsal head between the fingers and thumb of one hand and the adjacent head with the other hand, both thumbs being on the dorsum of the foot. Downward pressure on one metatarsal head, and upward pressure on the other, results in a small degree of movement. This small movement between the heads creates an even smaller, but definite, movement between the bases. If the lateral metatarsal head is taken in one hand and the metatarsal of the great toe is taken in the other, a considerable forward and backward movement is achieved due to combined movement of all metatarsal bases.

Although there is no contact between the two metatarsal heads, they are joined to each other by the powerful deep transverse metatarsal ligament. Occasionally this may become shortened; movement of one metatarsal head against its neighbour will help to mobilize this region.

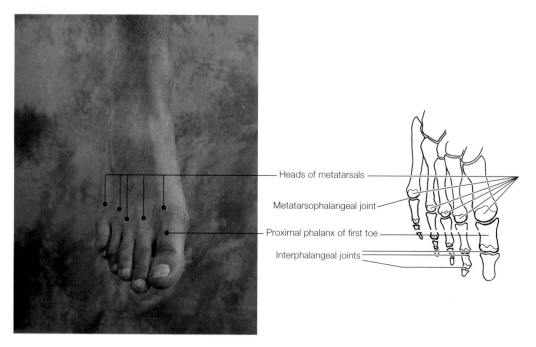

Fig. 3.11 (a), (b)
The metatarsophalangeal and interphalangeal joints of the right foot (dorsal aspect)

The metatarsophalangeal joints
[Figs 3.11 and 3.12]

These joints exist between the smooth, rounded heads of the metatarsal bones and the shallow cavity on the base of the proximal phalange. They are synovial condyloid joints, surrounded by a fairly loose capsule which is lined with synovial membrane. The articular surface on the head of the metatarsal extends onto its dorsal, distal and particularly plantar surfaces. The capsule is supported by cord-like collateral and strong plantar ligaments. A deep transverse metatarsal ligament links all the plantar ligaments together, forming a strong link between the heads of the metatarsals while allowing some up-and-down movement to occur between them.

Surface marking

The metatarsophalangeal joints lie on a line drawn from just distal to the head of the first metatarsal to just distal to the head of the fifth metatarsal. The line is slightly convex forward at its centre.

Palpation

Grip the **head of the first metatarsal** between your fingers and thumb. Let them slide slightly forwards. The joint space can easily be identified on the medial and dorsal aspect just distal to the head. Although the under-surface of the head is masked by a thick pad of fascia, the line of the joint can be traced with some difficulty.

If the lesser toes are strongly flexed, the heads of the metatarsals protrude on the dorsum of the foot. The joints can be palpated, with care, just beyond these heads. The tendons of extensor digitorum longus and brevis may have to be moved to the side. The joint of the fifth metatarsal can easily be palpated on its lateral side just beyond the head.

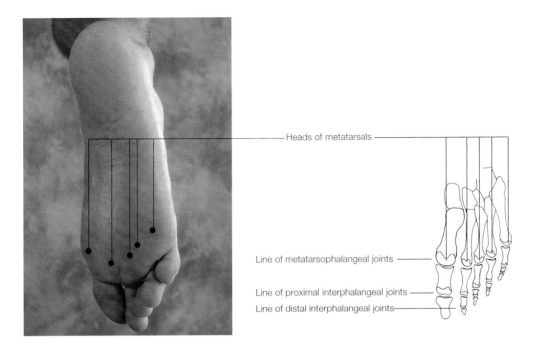

Fig. 3.11 (c), (d)
The metatarsophalangeal and interphalangeal joints of the right foot (plantar aspect)

With all the toes strongly extended, the joints can be identified from their plantar aspect but again they are partially masked by the thick fascia which covers them.

If the toes are rhythmically flexed and extended the proximal phalanges can be observed gliding over the heads of the metatarsals.

Accessory movements

These movements include rotation and a gliding of the proximal phalanx on the corresponding metatarsal head.

Grip the whole toe to be moved between the fingers and thumb of one hand, while stabilizing the remainder of the foot with the other. The toe can now be rotated about its long axis, and moved upwards, downwards and from side to side against the metatarsal head.

As in the case of many of the synovial joints with comparatively loose capsules, these joints can also be distracted, although not as much as the metacarpophalangeal joints of the hand and certainly not enough to cause the 'popping' sound that can be produced sometimes in the hand.

Stabilize the whole foot with one hand and grip the appropriate phalange with the fingers and thumb of the other. Now just apply a traction force on the phalange.

Although abduction and adduction is an active movement at these joints, it is often quite difficult to perform. This movement is easily obtainable, however, using the same technique as above and moving the phalange from side to side.

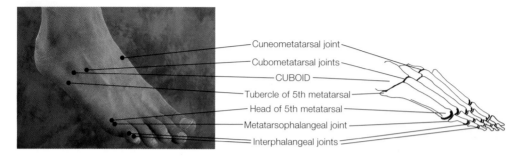

Fig. 3.12 (a), (b)
The metatarsophalangeal and interphalangeal joints of the right foot (lateral aspect)

The interphalangeal joints
[Figs 3.11 and 3.12]

These joints exit between the **proximal** and middle, and middle and **distal phalanges** of each of the lesser toes. As there are only **two phalanges** in the great toe, there is only one interphalangeal joint. These joints are synovial hinge joints surrounded by a capsule which is lined with synovial membrane and supp-orted by strong collateral and thick plantar ligaments. The plantar ligaments are composed of fibrocartilage and form part of the joint capsule.

At the distal end of each distal phalange the joint surface is replaced with the nail bed.

Palpation

On the second to fifth toes, the proximal interphal-angeal joints are usually flexed so that the head of the proximal phalanx is easy to palpate. In many subjects it is marked by a small bursa on its dorsal aspect. These joints can be palpated as a faint, horizontal line just beyond this bicondylar head, particularly if the middle phalanx is gripped between the finger and thumb and gently moved forwards and backwards. The joint is difficult to palpate on its plantar aspect. The distal interphalangeal joint is usually hyper-extended and, although the joint itself is difficult to feel, the movement available clearly marks its line, particularly when palpated from the plantar aspect (Figs 3.11c,d and 3.12).

The interphalangeal joint of the great toe can be palpated just beyond the head of the proximal phal-anx, particularly when the toe is flexed, and again can be emphasized by moving the distal phalanx for-wards and backwards in a similar fashion to the lesser toes (Fig. 3.11c,d).

Accessory movements

The interphalangeal joints are hinge joints. However, with the joint in slight flexion some side-to-side rocking of the joint can be produced.

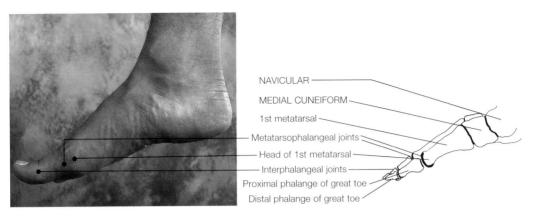

NAVICULAR
MEDIAL CUNEIFORM
1st metatarsal
Metatarsophalangeal joints
Head of 1st metatarsal
Interphalangeal joints
Proximal phalange of great toe
Distal phalange of great toe

Fig. 3.12 (c), (d)
The metatarsophalangeal and interphalangeal joints of the right foot (medial aspect)

Grasp the proximal of the two phalanges between finger and thumb of one hand and the more distal in a similar grip with the other hand. The distal phalanx can now be moved from side to side.

The joints of the foot are generally more difficult to mark and palpate. They are, however, all important in the functions of the foot, especially locomotion. Stiffness of just one small joint may lead to severe pain and dysfunction. It is therefore important to be able to locate and mobilize all joints, noting the direction of their articular surfaces and the resultant shape of the part as a whole.

All the joints of the foot, including the ankle, contribute to the overall position and shape of the foot. This will vary considerably according to its function at the time, i.e. weight-bearing or non-weight-bearing, mobile or stationary. It is therefore important to examine the structure in as many varying positions as possible.

In the standing position, weight transference through the foot is worthy of close examination. Body weight is transmitted through the tibia to the talus and then to the ground. The shape and position of the foot depend on where this downward force is applied to the arches and how the weight is distributed through the fore- and hind-foot to the ground. If the weight is applied too far to the medial side, the medial longitudinal arch becomes flattened, whereas if the weight is applied to the lateral side, the lateral longitudinal arch becomes flattened and the medial arch raised.

SELF-ASSESSMENT QUESTIONS

Page 58

1. Where does the zygapophyseal joint lie in relation to the spine of each lumbar vertebra?

Page 59

2. What is the only true accessory movement of the lumbar spine?

3. In which positions are these movements difficult to perform?

4. Why are they difficult to perform in these positions?

5. What methods of traction are available for the lumbar spine?

6. Describe one method of giving traction to the lumbar spine.

Page 62

7. List the surface markings of the pubic symphysis.

8. Describe the method by which the pubic symphysis can be palpated.

9. What movement occurs naturally at this joint?

10. Describe the method by which a possible accessory movement may be produced at the pubic symphysis.

11. How much movement is possible at this joint?

12. Under normal circumstances, is the sacroiliac joint more mobile in young or elderly people?

13. Is the joint more mobile in males or females?

Page 63

14. What is the posterior surface marking of the sacroiliac joint?

Page 64

15. Which surfaces take part in the sacroiliac joint?

16. Which accessory ligaments support the joint?

Please complete the labels below.

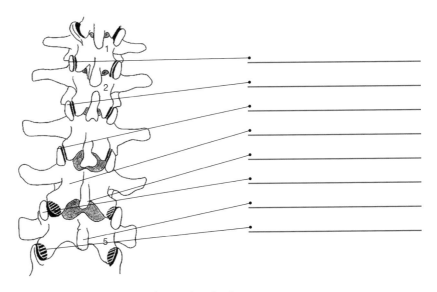

Fig. 3.1 (b) The zygapophyseal joints of the lumbar spine (posterior view)

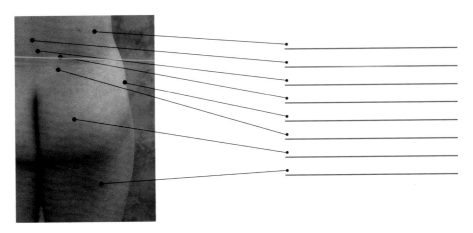

Fig. 3.3 (a) The right sacroiliac joint (posterior aspect)

Page 65

17. Give the class and type of this joint.

18. Name the ligaments supporting the joint.

19. Why is it advantageous to have a slightly mobile pelvis?

20. Which movement is considered to be a normal physiological movement of the sacrum?

21. Describe the way in which a slight accessory movement of this joint may be produced.

Page 66

22. What class and type is the hip joint?

23. How extensive is the synovial membrane of the hip joint?

24. Name the ligaments which support the capsule.

25. Which internal ligaments help to support the hip joint?

26. Which ligament attaches to the rim of the acetabulum?

27. What is the anterior surface marking of the hip joint?

28. Give the posterior surface markings of the hip joint.

Page 67

29. Explain the technique for palpating this joint.

30. List the accessory movements which may be produced at the hip joint.

Please complete the labels below.

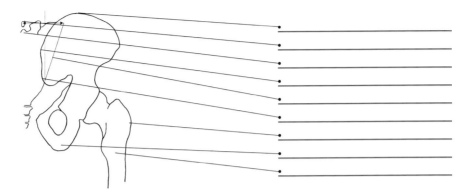

Fig. 3.3 (b) The right sacroiliac joint (posterior aspect)

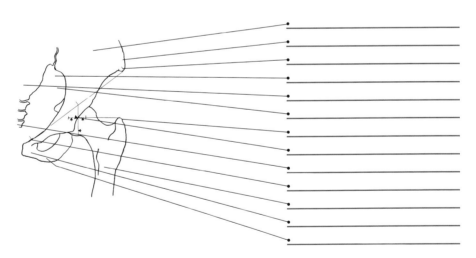

Fig. 3.4 (b) Bones of the left hip joint (anterior aspect)

Page 68

31. What is the class and type of the knee joint?
_____

32. Which bones take part in this joint?
_____

33. Describe the articular surfaces taking part in the knee joint.
_____

34. List the movements that occur at this joint.
_____

35. Describe the shape of the patella surface of the femur.
_____

36. Which structures form the anterior part of the capsule?
_____

37. Name the ligaments which support this joint externally.
_____

38. Which internal ligaments support the joint?
_____

39. Is this joint prone to dislocation?
_____

Page 69

40. What is the surface marking of the knee joint?
_____

41. Which structure can be palpated deep in the triangular spaces on either side of the ligamentum patellae?
_____

42. Explain how slight movement of these structures can be produced.
_____

43. Is it possible to palpate the knee joint from the posterior aspect?
_____

44. What term is used to describe the position of the knee in full extension?
_____

Page 70

45. Which accessory movements may be produced at the knee joint in the semiflexed position?
_____

46. List the factors that limit these movements.
_____

47. Which accessory movements can be produced at the patellofemoral joint when the knee is in full extension and the quadriceps muscles are relaxed?
_____

Page 71

48. If violent force is applied to the anterior surface of the upper part of the tibia, which of the cruciate ligaments is put under stress?
_____

49. Explain the mechanism by which the medial meniscus is usually damaged.
_____

Please complete the labels below.

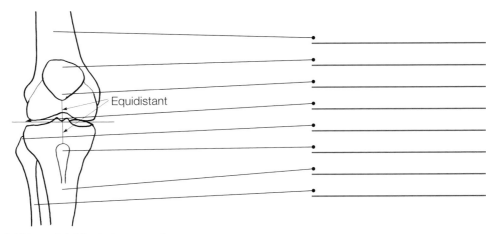

Fig. 3.5 (b) The right knee joint (anterior aspect)

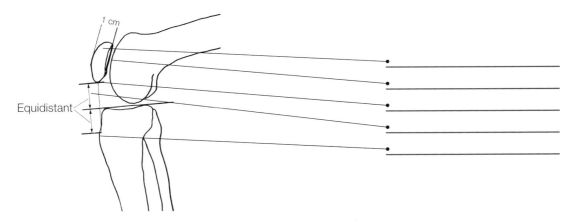

Fig. 3.5 (d) The right knee joint (medial aspect)

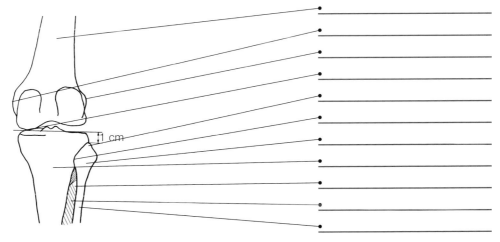

Fig. 3.5 (f) The right knee joint (posterior aspect)

Page 72

50. Name the joints which take place between the tibia and fibula.

51. What class and type is the superior tibiofibular joint?

52. Which ligaments support this joint?

53. What is the surface marking of the joint?

54. Which movement occurs at this joint during dorsiflexion and plantarflexion of the ankle joint?

55. Describe the accessory movements which can be performed at this joint.

Page 73

56. What is the class and type of the inferior tibiofibular joint?

57. What is the surface marking of this joint?

58. Name the very strong ligament which binds the two surfaces of the inferior joint together.

59. Which ligament of the inferior tibiofibular joint helps to form a socket for the ankle joint?

60. What structure binds the two shafts of the bones together?

61. In which direction do the fibres of this structure pass?

62. What term is used to describe the parting of the inferior tibiofibular joint caused by an injury? (fr)

Page 74

63. List the bones taking part in the ankle joint.

64. Describe the articular surfaces of these bones.

65. On which ligaments does the ankle joint depend for its stability?

66. Describe the extensive lower attachment of the ligament on the medial side of the joint.

67. What is the surface marking of the ankle joint?

Page 75

68. How much of this joint can be palpated?

69. Under what circumstances is the ankle joint described as 'close-packed'?

70. Which accessory movements can be produced at this joint and in what position?

Please complete the labels below.

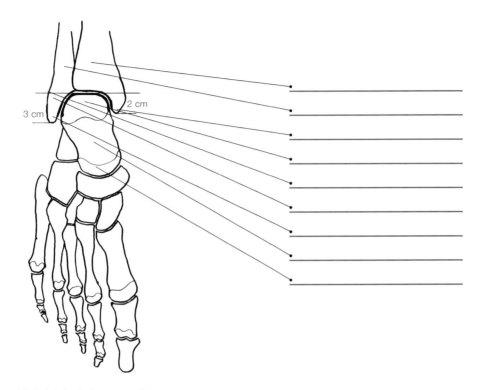

Fig. 3.7 (b) The right ankle joint (anterior aspect)

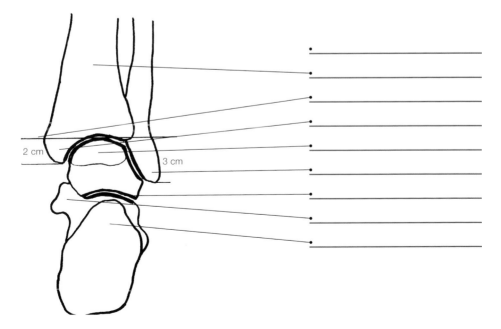

Fig. 3.7 (f) The right ankle joint (posterior aspect)

Page 78

71. List the different groups of joints in the foot.

72. Explain why it is difficult to palpate the joints of the foot from below.

73. Which surface of the talus takes part in the talocalcaneal joint?

74. Which surface of the calcaneus takes part in this joint?

75. On which ligaments does this joint rely for its support?

76. Describe the sinus tarsi.

77. What is the surface marking for the talocalcaneal joint?

78. Which surface of the sustentaculum tali is articular?

79. Name the bone which articulates with this surface.

Page 79

80. Which accessory movements may be produced at the talocalcaneal joint?

81. Describe the position of the hands used to obtain these movements.

Page 82

82. What is the class and type of the talocalcaneonavicular joint?

83. Which bony surfaces take part in this joint?

84. Name the ligaments which support the talocalcaneonavicular joint.

85. By what alternative name is the inferior ligament of this joint known?

86. What is the surface marking for the talocalcaneonavicular joint?

Page 83

87. How far, anteroinferiorly, is the tubercle of the navicular from the tip of the medial malleolus?

88. Which tendons may have to be moved aside to palpate the line of the joint?

89. Describe the accessory movements which can be produced at this joint.

Please complete the labels below.

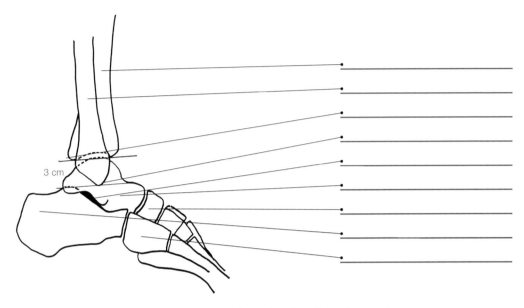

Fig. 3.8 (b) The talocalcaneal (subtalar) and ankle joint of the right foot (lateral aspect)

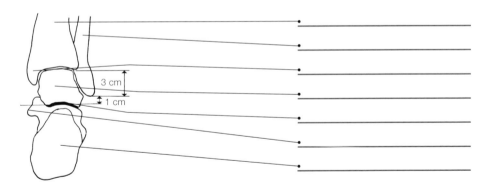

Fig. 3.8 (f) The talocalcaneal (subtalar) joint (posterior aspect)

Page 84

90. What is the classification and type of the calcaneocuboid joint?

91. Which surfaces take part in this joint?

92. Which ligaments support this joint?

93. What are the surface markings for the joint?

Page 85

94. Give the classification of the cuboideonavicular joint.

95. What is the surface marking of this joint?

96. List the joints which are involved in the midtarsal articulation.

97. What is the surface marking of this joint?

Page 86

98. What class and type are the cuneonavicular and intercuneiform joints?

99. Describe how the cuneiform bones are bound together distally.

100. With which structure do the three cuneiform bones articulate proximally?

101. How much movement occurs between the cuneiform bones?

Page 87

102. Which is the shortest of the three cuneiform bones?

103. Which metatarsal bone articulates with all three cuneiform bones?

104. With which bones do the 4th and 5th metatarsals articulate proximally?

105. Name the ligaments supporting these joints.

106. What is the surface marking of the tarsometatarsal joints?

Please complete the labels below.

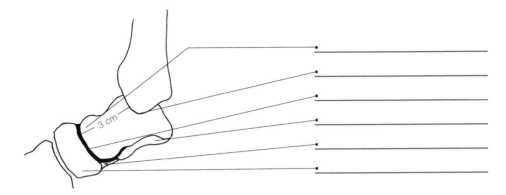

Fig. 3.9 (b) The talocalcaneonavicular joint of right foot (medial aspect)

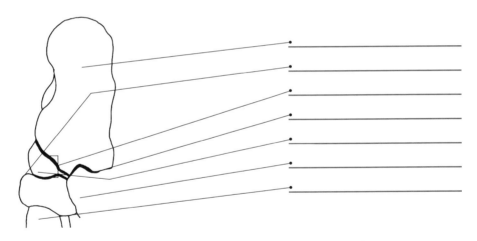

Fig. 3.9 (f) The talocalcaneonavicular and calcaneocuboid joint of right foot (plantar aspect)

Page 88

107. What is the classification and type of the intermetatarsal joints?

108. In which area are these joints located?

Page 89

109. Describe the way in which a limited amount of accessory movement can be produced at these joints.

110. What structure links the metatarsal heads together?

Page 90

111. What is the classification and type of the metatarsophalangeal joints?

112. Describe the articular surfaces taking part in these joints.

113. Name the ligaments which support these joints.

114. What are the surface markings of the metatarsophalangeal joints?

Page 91

115. Which accessory movements can be produced at these joints?

116. Name and describe a common deformity found at the first metatarsophalangeal joint. (fr)

Page 92

117. What is the classification and type of the interphalangeal joints?

118. Which ligaments support these joints?

119. Which accessory movements may be produced at these joints?

Page 93

120. Name and describe a common deformity found in the lesser toes. (fr)

121. Describe the way in which weight is distributed through the foot to the ground.

Please complete the labels below.

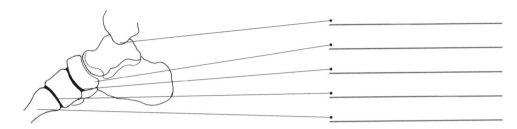

Fig. 3.9 (j) The cuneonavicular and cuneometatarsal joints of right foot (medial aspect)

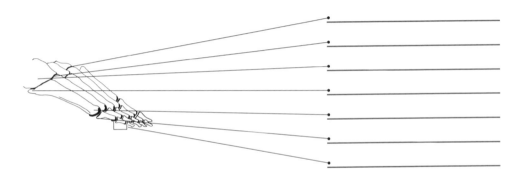

Fig. 3.12 (b) The metatarsophalangeal and interphalangeal joints of the right foot (lateral aspect)

Chapter 4
Muscles

Contents

The lateral and anterior aspect of the hip	110
Gluteus medius, gluteus minimus and tensor fasciae latae	110
Iliopsoas and pectineus	111
The posterior aspect of the hip and thigh	112
Gluteus maximus	112
The hamstrings	112
The anterior and medial aspects of the thigh	114
The adductors and quadriceps femoris	114
Sartorius	115
The anterior and lateral aspects of the lower leg and foot	116
Tibialis anterior	116
Extensor hallucis longus	116
Extensor digitorum longus	116
Peroneus tertius	117
Extensor digitorum brevis	117
The posterior and plantar aspects of the lower leg and foot	118
Popliteus	118
Triceps surae (calf)	118
Plantar muscles	120
Self-assessment questions	122

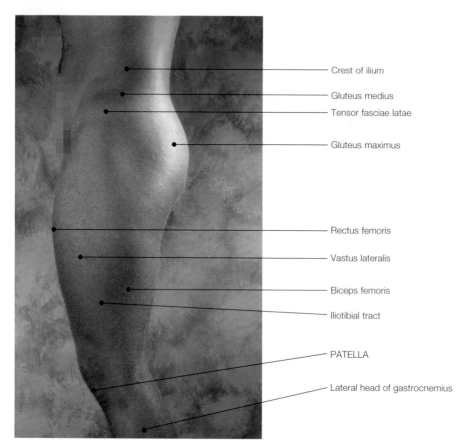

Crest of ilium

Gluteus medius

Tensor fasciae latae

Gluteus maximus

Rectus femoris

Vastus lateralis

Biceps femoris

Iliotibial tract

PATELLA

Lateral head of gastrocnemius

Fig. 4.1 (a)
Muscles of the left thigh
(lateral aspect)

THE LATERAL AND ANTERIOR ASPECT OF THE HIP

Gluteus medius, gluteus minimus and tensor fasciae latae

On the lateral aspect of the ilium, just anterior and deep to **gluteus maximus**, between the most lateral part of the **iliac crest** and the greater trochanter of the femur, gluteus medius can be located (Fig. 4.1a,b). It is covered by strong, thick fascia, but can, nevertheless, be felt contracting and relaxing when either, in standing, the weight is transferred from one leg to the other, the muscle preventing the pelvis dropping to the opposite side, or, in side lying, when the limb is raised and lowered. Anterior to gluteus medius, the bulk of gluteus minimus, covered by the tensor fasciae latae (Fig. 4.1a,b), is readily palpable between the anterior section of the iliac crest and the **greater trochanter**. The contraction of these two muscles is produced in lying or standing when the foot is medially rotated, as in the weight-bearing phase of walking when the lower limb is moving into extensi-

on and medial rotation, just before the thrust phase produced by the **gastrocnemius**.

It is important to practise the palpation of these muscles, gluteus maximus, medius, minimus and tensor fasciae latae, in the subject or patient during ambulation. Much information can be gained from this region regarding the relationships of the bony structures and the power and timing of muscle contraction. As noted above, the gluteus medius should contract on the weight-bearing limb to prevent the pelvis dropping to the other side when the foot is raised from the ground. Therefore, the distance between the iliac crest and the greater trochanter of the femur, on the weight-bearing limb, should remain the same or even decrease slightly.

It is also worth noting, through palpation of these muscles, that as the weight-bearing limb moves from

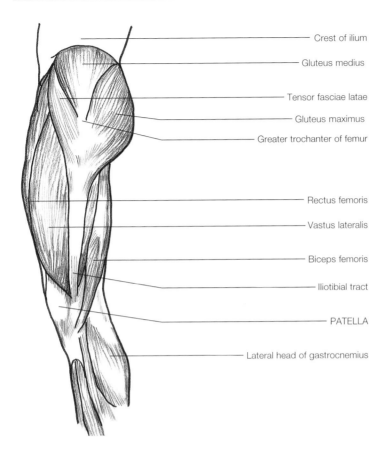

Fig. 4.1 (b)
Muscles of the left thigh
(lateral aspect)

the flexed to the extended position, the muscles appear to contract in sequence from posterior to anterior. As the heel comes in contact with the ground, the limb is in lateral rotation and the posterior section of gluteus medius and possibly gluteus maximus are contracted. As the hip moves forwards over the foot, the middle of gluteus medius can be felt contracting, and as the limb moves into extension and medial rotation, the anterior section of gluteus medius, gluteus minimus and tensor fasciae latae are contracted. During this sequence, the pelvis will rotate around the weight-bearing hip joint towards the weight-bearing side. Finally, it is worth noting that immediately the limb is weight-bearing, the gluteus medius contracts.

Dysfunction of the hip joint may upset the precise *firing off* of these muscles.

Iliopsoas and pectineus

The front of the hip joint is crossed by iliopsoas and pectineus, the former being a broad tendon and the latter a quadrilateral muscle. Because they are both covered by several layers of fascia, as well as the femoral sheath and its contents, they are difficult to palpate (see Fig. 4.3a,b).

Palpation

With the subject lying supine and both the hip and knee supported and flexed to 90°, place your fingers on the anterior aspect of the hip joint 3.5 cm below the centre of the inguinal ligament. If the subject now gently flexes and extends the hip joint, the contraction of both iliopsoas laterally and pectineus medially can be palpated.

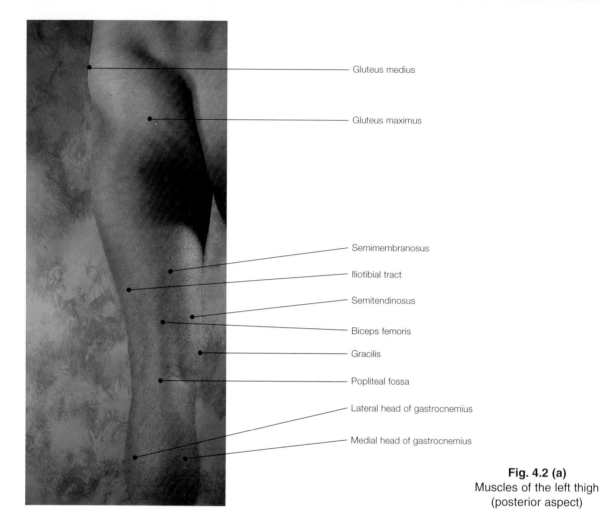

Gluteus medius

Gluteus maximus

Semimembranosus

Iliotibial tract

Semitendinosus

Biceps femoris

Gracilis

Popliteal fossa

Lateral head of gastrocnemius

Medial head of gastrocnemius

Fig. 4.2 (a)
Muscles of the left thigh
(posterior aspect)

THE POSTERIOR ASPECT OF THE HIP AND THIGH

Gluteus maximus

The extremely well-developed muscles around the hip joint are the gluteal muscles, especially the **gluteus maximus**, which is important in maintaining the upright posture. It is a large and powerful muscle, giving the gluteal region its rounded shape.

Gluteus maximus (Figs 4.1 and 4.2) lies between the posterior part of the iliac crest superiorly, the anal cleft medially and the gluteal fold inferiorly. With care, its coarse fibres can be traced running downwards and laterally towards the greater trochanter of the femur. It is often possible, especially with the hip extended, to trace the more superficial fibres to their attachment into the fascia lata (**iliotibial tract**). The extent of the muscle is made clearer if the subject extends the hip when lying prone.

The hamstrings

Below the gluteal fold the hamstrings are evident. These powerful muscles cover the whole of the back of the thigh. **Semitendinosus** and **semimembranosus** pass downwards and medially, with the **biceps** crossing to lie laterally as it passes down to the knee. The muscle bellies of the hamstrings separate approximately two-thirds of the way down the thigh, giving rise to their tendons – semitendinosus and semimembranosus medially and **biceps femoris** laterally (Fig. 4.2).

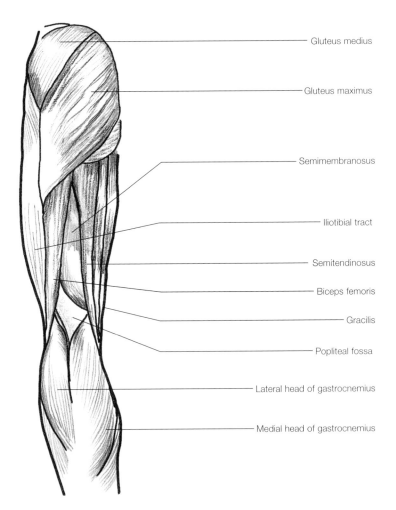

Gluteus medius

Gluteus maximus

Semimembranosus

Iliotibial tract

Semitendinosus

Biceps femoris

Gracilis

Popliteal fossa

Lateral head of gastrocnemius

Medial head of gastrocnemius

Fig. 4.2 (b)
Muscles of the left thigh
(posterior aspect)

Palpation

With the subject lying prone and flexing the knee against resistance, the tendon of biceps femoris stands clear on the posterolateral side of the knee, and can be traced to its insertion to the head of the fibula. Proximally the superficial fusiform muscle belly can be followed towards the ischial tuberosity (see Fig. 2.3). The deeper fibres of biceps femoris can be palpated on the medial side of the tendon in the upper part of the **popliteal fossa**. The tendon of semitendinosus can be observed, and palpated, on the posteromedial side of the knee joint as it passes downwards to its attachment on the medial surface of the tibial condyle and shaft. Proximally, its fusiform muscle belly joins that of biceps femoris near the gluteal fold. A slightly thinner tendon, lying anteromedial, can be identified.

This is the tendon of **gracilis** whose muscle belly can be traced up the medial side of the thigh as far as the body of the pubis, particularly when the knee is flexed against resistance. Semimembranosus lies deep to semitendinosus just above the knee. It is difficult to palpate, even at its distal end, because it attaches, via a broad aponeurosis, to the postero-medial aspect of the medial condyle of the tibia.

With the knee supported in approximately 60° of flexion, press your fingertips and thumb into the space on either side of the semitendinosus tendon approximately 5 cm above the level of the knee joint. As the subject gently flexes and extends the knee, the muscle below can be felt contracting and then relaxing.

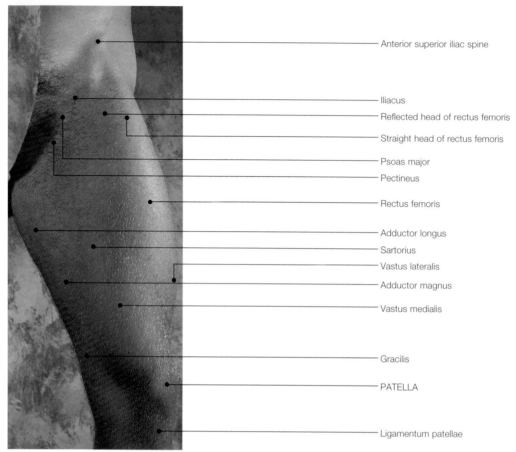

- Anterior superior iliac spine
- Iliacus
- Reflected head of rectus femoris
- Straight head of rectus femoris
- Psoas major
- Pectineus
- Rectus femoris
- Adductor longus
- Sartorius
- Vastus lateralis
- Adductor magnus
- Vastus medialis
- Gracilis
- PATELLA
- Ligamentum patellae

Fig. 4.3 (a)
Muscles of the left thigh
(medial aspect)

THE ANTERIOR AND MEDIAL ASPECTS OF THE THIGH

The adductors and quadriceps femoris

If the thigh is now adducted, the adductor group of muscles comes into action. The following can be palpated: the tendinous part of **adductor magnus** running down the medial aspect of the thigh from the ischial tuberosity to the **adductor tubercle, adductor longus** lying anteriorly and laterally with adductor brevis and the aponeurotic part of adductor magnus lying more posteriorly. However, it is difficult to identify the adductor muscles separately.

The great bulk of muscle on the front of the thigh is the quadriceps femoris, consisting of **vastus medialis, vastus intermedius, vastus lateralis** and **rectus femoris**. It extends from the anterior inferior iliac spine and above the acetabulum (the attachment of the rectus femoris) via the **patella** to the **tibial tuberosity** (Fig. 4.3).

Palpation

Three of the four bellies of quadriceps femoris can readily be palpated when the knee is extended against resistance. The belly of the vastus intermedius lies deep to the other three and is difficult to identify separately.

Rectus femoris passes straight down the front of the thigh from the anterior inferior iliac spine to the base of the patella. Its proximal and distal tendons can clearly be identified. Its belly appears as a fusiform shape on the front of the thigh.

The belly of **vastus lateralis** can be identified halfway down the lateral surface of the thigh, being flattened posteriorly by the fascia lata iliotibial tract (see Fig. 4.1).

Vastus medialis can be identified on the medial side of the thigh just above the level of the patella. It

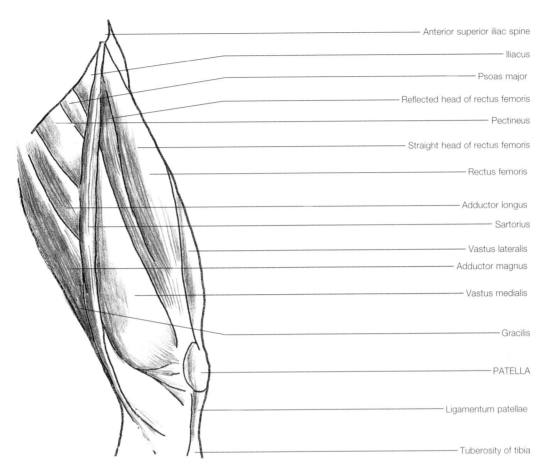

Anterior superior iliac spine

Iliacus

Psoas major

Reflected head of rectus femoris

Pectineus

Straight head of rectus femoris

Rectus femoris

Adductor longus

Sartorius

Vastus lateralis

Adductor magnus

Vastus medialis

Gracilis

PATELLA

Ligamentum patellae

Tuberosity of tibia

Fig. 4.3 (b)
Muscles of the left thigh
(medial aspect)

varies considerably in size according to its use and is the first part of the quadriceps to show signs of weakness. Its lowest fibres can be traced running almost horizontally and laterally to attach to the medial border of the patella.

The tendon of the quadriceps, particularly of rectus femoris and vastus intermedius, can be identified attaching to the upper border of the patella. There are often small depressions on its medial and lateral edges where it joins the expansion of vastus lateralis and vastus medialis. The patella is a sesamoid bone and lies within the tendon of quadriceps femoris, the **ligamentum patellae** being a continuation of the quadriceps tendon (Fig. 4.3). The ligamentum patellae joins the apex of the patella to the upper part of the tibial tuberosity. It is approximately 5 cm long and 2 cm wide, with its central point level with the knee joint (see pages 69 and 71). When the knee is fully extended, a strong tendon-like structure can be palpated lying

lateral to the patella and running down to attach to the lateral tibial condyle (Fig. 4.4a,b). This is the lower part of the iliotibial tract, and can be traced superiorly along the lateral side of the thigh to the ilium.

Sartorius

With the subject lying supine, resist the movement of flexion, lateral rotation, abduction of the hip and flexion of the knee by applying resistance to the heel. The long strap-like **sartorius** muscle can be observed and palpated, crossing the thigh from the **anterior superior iliac spine** above to the medial condyle of the tibia below (Fig. 4.3). Its upper third appears to stand away from the groin region. With the subject sitting with the knees extended, contraction of both muscles simultaneously produces the 'tailor sitting' position. Sartorius [*sartor* (L) = tailor] can be observed and palpated during this action.

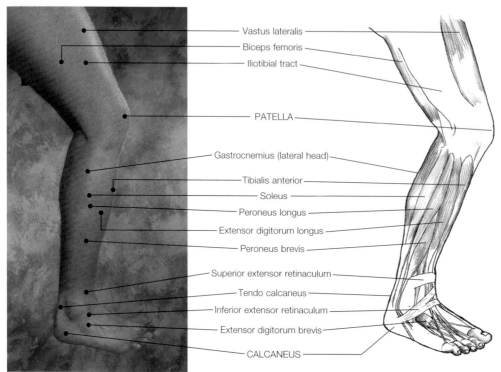

Vastus lateralis
Biceps femoris
Iliotibial tract

PATELLA

Gastrocnemius (lateral head)
Tibialis anterior
Soleus
Peroneus longus
Extensor digitorum longus
Peroneus brevis
Superior extensor retinaculum
Tendo calcaneus
Inferior extensor retinaculum
Extensor digitorum brevis
CALCANEUS

Fig. 4.4 (a), (b)
Muscles of the right leg
(lateral aspect)

THE ANTERIOR AND LATERAL ASPECTS OF THE LOWER LEG AND FOOT

The muscles in the anterior compartment of the leg are relatively superficial and are easy to identify. Even so, differentiation is easiest where the tendons pass over the front of the ankle joint and palpation should begin here.

Tibialis anterior

With the subject lying supine and the foot dorsiflexed, find the most medial tendon, that of **tibialis anterior** (Fig. 4.4). Although it lies deep to the **superior** and **inferior extensor retinacula**, it is clear to see and feel. Distally it can be traced to its insertion on the medial cuneiform and base of the first metatarsal. Proximally, the strong tendon gives way to a firm but narrow muscle which fills the space lateral to the anterior border of the tibia. The muscle is contained within strong fascia and becomes particularly hard on contraction. There is often a narrow space between the muscle and the tibia anteriorly.

Extensor hallucis longus

The tendon lying lateral to tibialis anterior at the ankle joint is that of **extensor hallucis longus** (Fig. 4.4c,d). It also stands clear of the joint and can be traced across the medial side of the foot to the great toe where, if the toe is extended, it can be followed to its insertion into the base of the distal phalanx. Proximally, the tendon is soon lost between the other muscles; however, if the line of the tendon is continued to the middle of the fibula, the muscle can be felt contracting deep to extensor digitorum longus.

Extensor digitorum longus

Lateral to the tendon of extensor hallucis longus lies the tendon of **extensor digitorum longus** (Fig. 4.4a–d). Immediately distal to the ankle it can be seen dividing into four separate tendons, which can be traced to the dorsal surface of the lateral four toes. Occasionally, when the toes are flexed at the metatarsophalangeal joint, the tendons can be felt and seen to 'bowstring' across the joint. Proximally, the tendon soon becomes

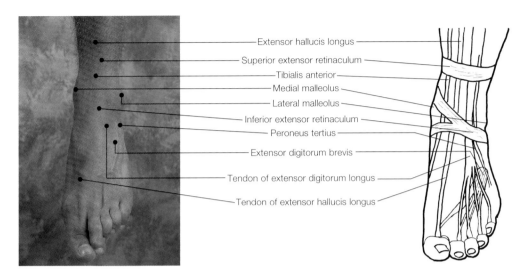

Fig. 4.4 (c), (d)
Tendons and muscles of the left foot
(dorsal aspect)

Extensor hallucis longus
Superior extensor retinaculum
Tibialis anterior
Medial malleolus
Lateral malleolus
Inferior extensor retinaculum
Peroneus tertius
Extensor digitorum brevis
Tendon of extensor digitorum longus
Tendon of extensor hallucis longus

muscular, extending superiorly as far as the superior tibiofibular joint, lying between tibialis anterior medially and the fibula laterally.

Peroneus tertius

Although this small muscle is named as one of the peroneal muscles, **peroneus tertius** is considered to be part of the extensor digitorum longus, in fact its fifth tendon. This may be borne out as it does arise from the lower third of the fibula in line with, and does pass under, the superior extensor retinaculum and through the loop of the inferior retinaculum, with, and lateral to, the extensor digitorum longus. However, unlike the extensor digitorum longus, it does not insert into the digits but into the medial side of the dorsal surface of the base of the fifth metatarsal. In a small percentage of subjects the muscle is absent.

The tendon of the peroneus tertius is difficult to find, but is best located as it crosses the lateral part of the dorsum of the foot on its way to attach to the

medial side of the base of the fifth metatarsal (Fig. 4.4c,d).

Palpation

From the base of the fifth metatarsal, draw a line from its medial side towards the lower quarter of the shaft of the fibula. It is along this line that the tendon is most likely to be palpated, particularly when the foot is everted.

Extensor digitorum brevis

Extensor digitorum brevis presents as a large swelling some 2 cm anterior to the lateral malleolus on the dorsolateral aspect of the foot (Fig. 4.4). Four narrow tendons can be palpated, leaving its distal aspect passing towards the medial four toes. In the second, third and fourth toes the tendons join those of extensor digitorum longus, while in the great toe the tendon passes to the lateral side of the proximal phalanx.

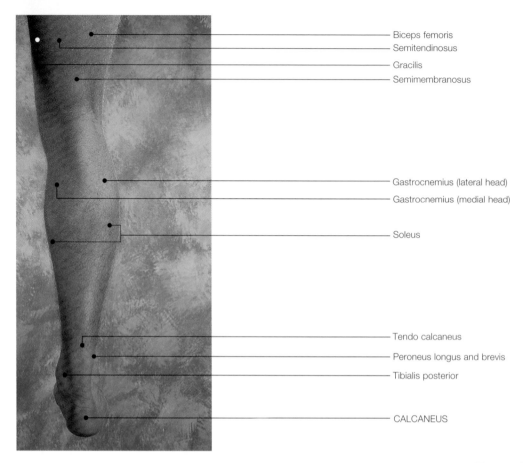

- Biceps femoris
- Semitendinosus
- Gracilis
- Semimembranosus

- Gastrocnemius (lateral head)
- Gastrocnemius (medial head)

- Soleus

- Tendo calcaneus
- Peroneus longus and brevis
- Tibialis posterior

- CALCANEUS

Fig. 4.5 (a)
Muscles of the right leg and foot
(posterior aspect)

THE POSTERIOR AND PLANTAR ASPECTS OF THE LOWER LEG AND FOOT

Popliteus

Popliteus lies deep within the **popliteal fossa** high up on the posterolateral aspect of the knee joint. Its tendon, however, can be palpated as it passes below the lateral epicondyle of the femur. With the subject sitting and the knee flexed 90°, place the tips of your fingers on the lateral surface of the femoral condyle just below and in front of the lateral epicondyle. If medial rotation of the leg at the knee joint is now performed, the tendon of popliteus can be palpated as it runs forwards, in a groove, towards its femoral attachment.

Triceps surae (calf)

The posterior aspect of the leg is dominated by the beautifully shaped calf muscles **gastrocnemius** and **soleus**, the former being more superficial and the latter deep. Together they are attached distally by the tendo calcaneus to the posterior surface of the **calcaneus**. The two muscles, however, arise from different bones. The gastrocnemius from the femur, its medial head from the upper part of the medial condyle and the lateral head from just above the lateral epicondyle. The soleus, which is believed to derive its name from a flat fish, the sole, arises below the knee joint from the posterior surfaces of the tibia, fibula and interosseous membrane.

Plantaris, when present, passes lateral to medial, from the upper part of the lateral condyle of the femur downwards, between gastrocnemius and soleus to attach adjacent to the tendo calcaneus.

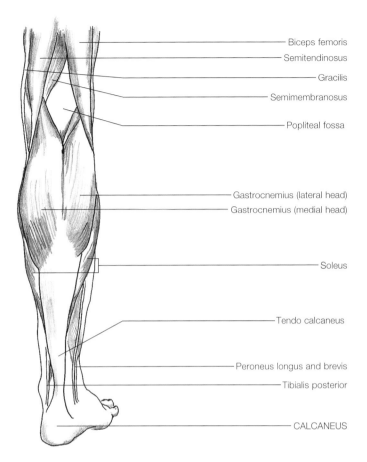

Fig. 4.5 (b)
Muscles of the right leg and foot
(posterior aspect)

Palpation

With the subject standing, begin at the posterior aspect of the heel, where the broad tendo calcaneus can easily be identified attaching to the calcaneus. Follow the tendon upwards for some 8 cm as it narrows to a width of approximately 1 cm, after which it rapidly widens into an aponeurosis about 8 cm wide. Here the muscle fibres of gastrocnemius can be palpated attaching to the superficial surface of the aponeurosis. Two large bellies, the medial and longer belly, stretch to the medial femoral condyle, and the lateral belly to the lateral femoral condyle (Fig. 4.5). The two bellies are separated by a faint vertical line which is easily palpable in a well-developed calf.

Soleus lies deep to gastrocnemius, its fibres contributing to the deep surface of the **tendo calcaneus**. Its upper attachment is to the posterior aspect of the tibia (soleal line) and to the head and shaft of the fibula. The muscle belly is broad and thick. As soleus is

primarily a postural muscle, preventing the tibia from tilting forwards in the standing position, it is easier to palpate when the subject is standing.

First locate the broad aponeurosis of the tendo calcaneus where it joins the muscle fibres of gastrocnemius, and run your fingers to the outer borders. Immediately adjacent is the muscle belly of soleus bulging either side and deep to the aponeurosis (Fig. 4.5). If the subject gently raises the heel, the muscle fibres of gastrocnemius can be felt contracting.

If the subject then fully flexes the knee and plantarflexes the foot, soleus can be felt contracting while gastrocnemius remains relaxed. This is because the upper (femoral) and lower (calcaneal) attachments of gastrocnemius are brought closer together, shortening the muscle and essentially preventing it from contracting. This is known as 'muscle insufficiency'.

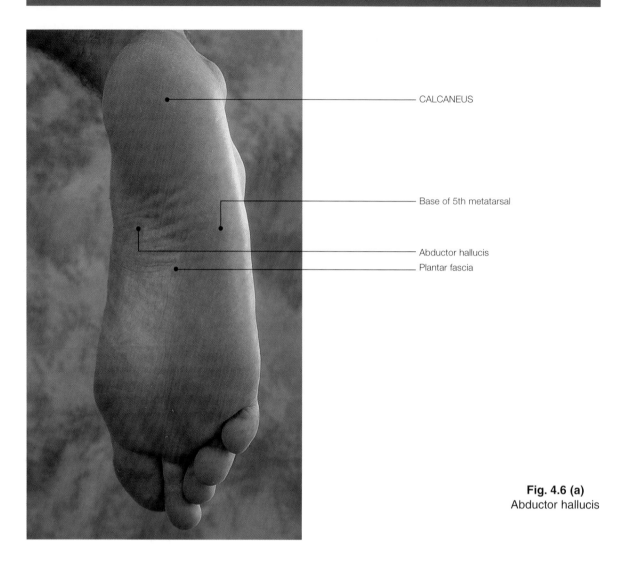

CALCANEUS

Base of 5th metatarsal

Abductor hallucis
Plantar fascia

Fig. 4.6 (a)
Abductor hallucis

Plantar muscles [Fig. 4.6]

The plantar surface of the foot is covered centrally by a thick dense layer of **fascia** known as the **plantar aponeurosis**. This is triangular in shape, being narrower posteriorly, where it attaches to the **calcaneus**, and broader anteriorly, where it splits to attach either side of the **proximal phalanx** of each toe. It gives the central portion of the plantar aspect a pale appearance, the heel, lateral border and under the metatarsal heads being darker and covered with harder skin for weight-bearing.

The plantar muscles are arranged in four layers deep to the plantar fascia, and are relatively easily recognized on dissection. The deepest muscles are the shortest, whereas those just deep to the plantar aponeurosis are the longest. All of these muscles except **abductor hallucis** are difficult to palpate due to the thickness and tension of the fascia.

Palpation

Only abductor hallucis is easily recognizable on the medial side of the foot. Some subjects may be able to abduct their great toe, in which case the belly of abductor hallucis can be palpated along the medial border of the foot. The broad fusiform-shaped muscle belly passes forwards from the medial tubercle of the calcaneus, continuing as a tendon to the medial side of the proximal phalange of the great toe.

If the subject is unable to abduct the great toe (really more of a party trick than anything else), shortening the foot while weight-bearing produces a powerful contraction of the muscle. This is most probably the muscle's main functional activity. The bulk of the muscle is palpated in its posterior section, with the relatively thick tendon distinct in its anterior half

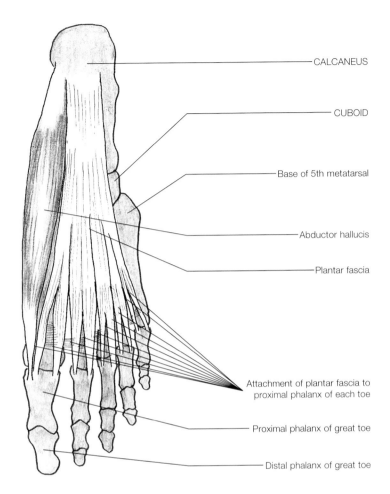

CALCANEUS

CUBOID

Base of 5th metatarsal

Abductor hallucis

Plantar fascia

Attachment of plantar fascia to
proximal phalanx of each toe

Proximal phalanx of great toe

Distal phalanx of great toe

Fig. 4.6 (b)
Abductor hallux and plantar fascia of the right foot
(plantar aspect)

inserting into the medial side of the base of the proximal phalanx of the great toe. If the toe is extended, the
medial edge of the plantar fascia can be palpated as it
is being stretched.

The use and type of footwear, if any, habitually worn,
together with the activities and weight of the subject,
will influence the structure and appearance of the foot.
There is usually a thickening of the fascia and hardening
of the skin over weight-bearing areas, these normally
being over the heel, lateral border of the foot and heads
of the metatarsals, particularly the first and fifth.

The amount of the sole of the foot which is in
contact with the supporting surface is inversely proportional to the height of the plantar arches. The
medial side of the foot is rarely in contact with the
ground, except in subjects with extremely flat feet.
Anteriorly, the metatarsal heads are normally in contact with the ground and may show a downward
convexity, producing areas of hardened skin (callus),
under the second, third and fourth metatarsal heads.

SELF-ASSESSMENT QUESTIONS

Page 110

1. Describe the location of the gluteus medius.

2. In what area of the body can its contraction be felt?

3. What tissue covers the gluteus medius?

4. Give the attachments of this muscle proximally. (fr)

5. Where does it attach inferiorly? (fr)

6. In standing, which gluteus medius muscle contracts strongly when the left leg is raised from the floor?

7. Which two muscles lie anterior to the gluteus medius?

8. How can these two muscles be brought into action?

Page 111

9. When the weight-bearing lower limb is moving from flexion to extension, in which direction does the hip joint rotate?

10. How may dysfunction of the hip joint affect the surrounding muscles? (fr)

11. Which two muscles pass across the anterior aspect of the hip joint?

12. Explain why these two muscles are difficult to palpate.

13. Describe a technique whereby these muscles may be palpated.

14. Name one structure that lies in front of these muscles.

Page 112

15. In which area of the body is the gluteus maximus muscle located?

16. Name an important function of the gluteus maximus.

17. For which type of fibres is this muscle particularly noted?

18. In which direction do these fibres pass?

19. Where does the gluteus maximus muscle attach distally?

Please complete the labels below.

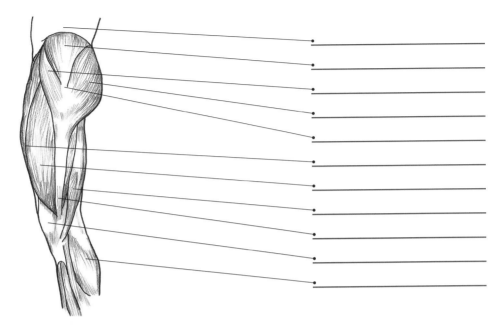

Fig. 4.1 (b) Muscles of the left thigh (lateral aspect)

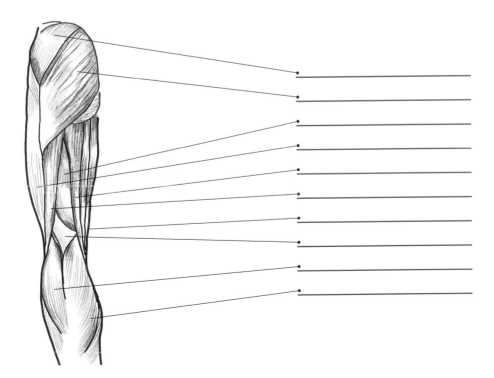

Fig. 4.2 (b) Muscles of the left thigh (posterior aspect)

20. Describe the way in which this muscle may be put into action.

21. In which area of the body are the hamstring muscles located?

22. List the muscles which comprise the hamstrings.

23. Which of these muscles pass downwards and medially?

24. Name the hamstring muscle which passes downwards and laterally.

25. How far down the thigh do the bellies of the hamstrings separate?

Page 113

26. Describe a technique for palpating these muscles.

27. Describe the distal attachment of the biceps femoris.

28. To what prominence of which bone do these muscles attach proximally?

29. In which area can the deeper fibres, from the short head, of the biceps femoris be palpated?

30. Describe where the tendon of the semitendinosus can be palpated.

31. Where does the tendon of the semitendinosus attach distally?

32. With which muscle does the semitendinosus blend proximally?

33. Name the muscle which has the thin tendon lying anteromedial to the tendon of semitendinosus.

34. Where does this thin muscle attach proximally?

35. Explain why the semimembranosus is difficult to palpate.

36. Where does semimembranosus attach distally?

37. What structure is given support by the fibrous lower attachment of semimembranosus? (fr)

38. Describe the way in which the semimembranosus can be palpated.

Please complete the labels below.

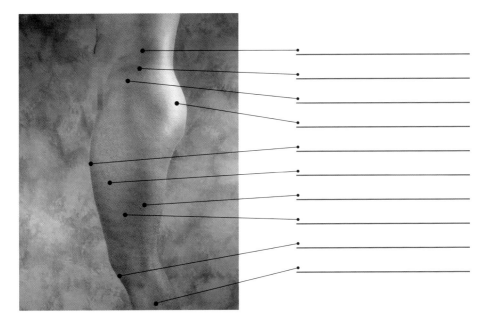

Fig. 4.1 (a) Muscles of the left thigh (lateral aspect)

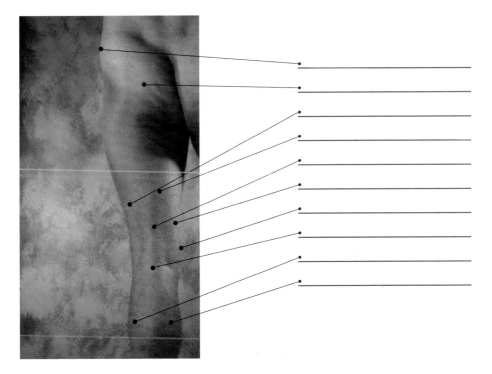

Fig. 4.2 (a) Muscles of the left thigh (posterior aspect)

Page 114

39. Which main muscle group is located on the medial aspect of the thigh?

40. List the muscles which comprise the medial group.

41. Where does the tendinous section of the largest muscle of the above group attach, distally?

42. What is the collective name of the main muscle group which forms the anterior aspect of the thigh?

43. From medial to lateral, list the muscles of the anterior group.

44. Where does the rectus femoris attach proximally?

45. What name is given to the section of the quadriceps tendon below the patella?

46. Where does this section of the quadriceps tendon attach distally?

47. Which three quadriceps muscles can be easily palpated?

48. Which structure flattens the lateral muscle of this group?

Page 115

49. Which is the lowest of the three quadriceps muscle bellies?

50. Following an injury, which of the quadriceps muscles usually atrophies first?

51. Name the two tendons which attach to the base of the patella.

52. What type of bone is the patella?

53. Under normal circumstances, how long is the ligamentum patellae?

54. Explain its relevance to the surface marking of the knee joint.

55. Name the tendon-like structure lying lateral to the patella when the knee is extended.

56. To what is this structure attached distally?

57. Where does the sartorius muscle attach proximally?

58. What is its attachment distally?

59. List the actions performed by the sartorius muscle.

60. Describe the position which results from its action.

61. What is the derivation of the name 'sartorius'?

Please complete the labels below.

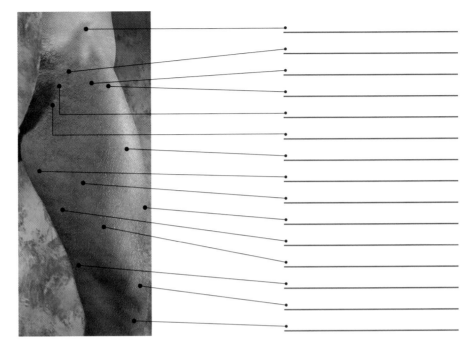

Fig. 4.3 (a) Muscles of the left thigh (medial aspect)

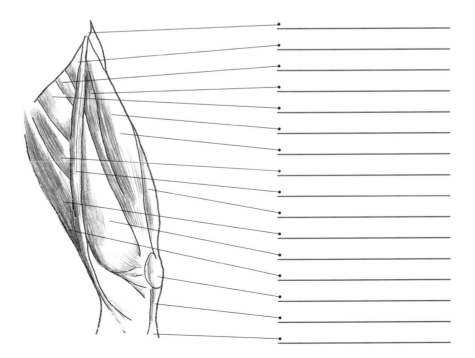

Fig. 4.3 (b) Muscles of the left thigh (medial aspect)

Page 116

62. List the muscles located in the anterior compartment of the leg.

63. Which is the most medial tendon, anteriorly, when the ankle joint is dorsiflexed?

64. Name the structure, beneath which this tendon passes, as it crosses the ankle joint.

65. Where does this muscle insert distally?

66. Which structure lies medial to the belly of this muscle?

67. Which tendon lies lateral to the above tendon?

68. What is the distal insertion of this tendon?

69. In which area can this muscle be felt contracting?

70. Which muscle tendon lies lateral to that of the extensor hallucis muscle?

71. Describe what happens to this tendon just below the level of the ankle joint.

Page 117

72. What is the peroneus tertius considered to be?

73. With which muscle does peroneus tertius pass through the loop of the extensor retinaculum?

74. Where does peroneus tertius insert distally?

75. What action is produced by this muscle?

76. Where is the extensor digitorum brevis muscle located?

77. Towards which four toes do the tendons pass?

78. Describe how these tendons differ in their insertion.

Page 118

79. Where in the body is the popliteus muscle situated?

80. Where can its tendon be located?

81. Describe how the popliteus muscle may be put into action.

82. By what other name is the calf muscle also known?

Please complete the labels below.

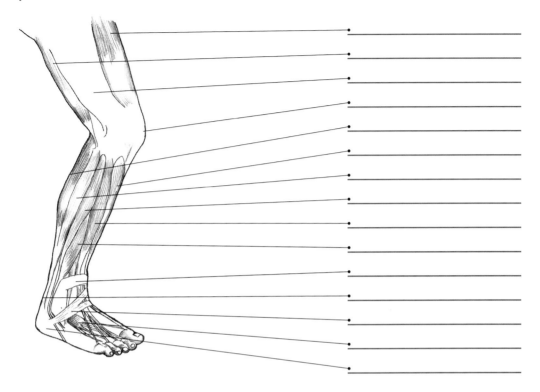

Fig. 4.4 (b) Muscles of the right leg (lateral aspect)

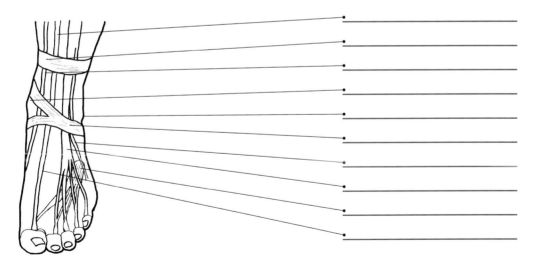

Fig. 4.4 (d) Tendons and muscles of the left foot (dorsal aspect)

83. List the muscles which comprise this group.

_____

84. Which muscle is more superficial than the others?

_____

85. Describe their attachment to the calcaneus.

86. Describe the attachment of the proximal end of the most superficial muscle.

87. What is the proximal attachment of the deepest of this muscle group?

88. Which muscle passes between the two?

89. Approximately, how long is the tendo calcaneus?

90. How wide is it at its widest point?

91. Describe the muscular form of the most superficial muscle of the group.

Page 119

92. Under what conditions is it easiest to palpate the deepest muscle of this group?

93. In what area can the deepest muscle be palpated?

94. Describe a technique for putting the calf muscles into action.

95. Explain how a contraction of the deepest muscle can be obtained while achieving a simultaneous relaxation of the most superficial muscle.

Page 120

96. Which structure covers the central area of the plantar aspect of the foot?

97. Describe the shape of this structure.

98. Where does it attach posteriorly?

99. What is its anterior attachment?

100. Describe the general arrangement of the plantar muscles of the foot.

101. Which of these muscles is palpable?

102. In which area is this muscle palpated?

Page 121

103. Where does this muscle attach posteriorly?

104. What is its attachment anteriorly?

105. List the actions of this muscle.

Please complete the labels below.

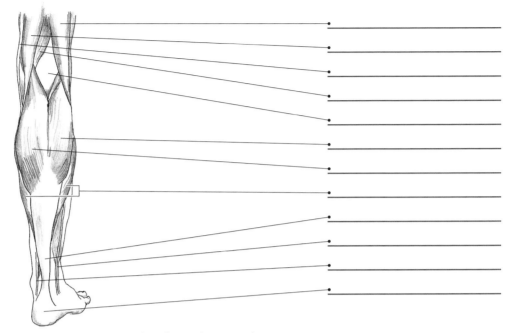

Fig. 4.5 (b) Muscles of the right leg and foot (posterior aspect)

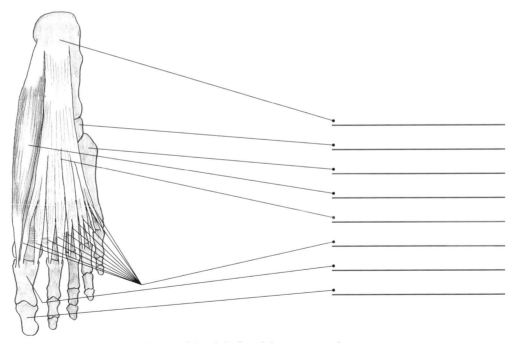

Fig. 4.6 (b) Abductor hallux and plantar fascia of the right foot (plantar aspect)

106. Under normal circumstances, in which area is the hardest skin of the plantar aspect of the foot located?

_____

Chapter 5
Nerves

Contents

Sciatic nerve and its derivatives   134
Self-assessment questions   136

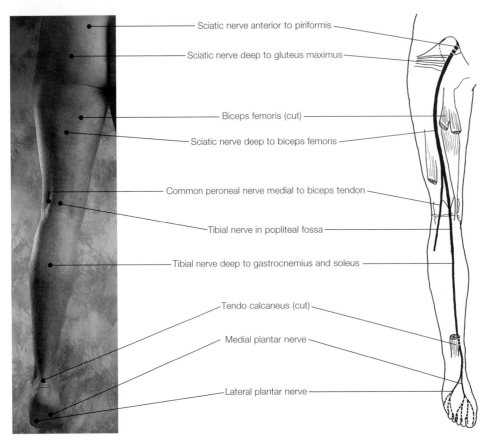

Fig. 5.1 (a), (b)
The sciatic nerve and branches in the left lower limb (posterior view)

The nerves of the lower limb are normally deep within the tissues and thus extremely difficult to palpate. Nevertheless, it is important to be aware of their location and to be able to palpate those that venture close to the surface.

The whole of the lower limb is supplied from the lumbar, sacral and coccygeal plexi. The lumbar plexus derives its fibres from T12, L1, L2, L3 and L4 roots. The sacral (lumbosacral) plexus derives its fibres from L4, L5, S1, S2, S3 and S4. The coccygeal (sacral) plexus derives its fibres from S4 and S5. These form a complex arrangement of nerves, most of which are not palpable, but nevertheless remain essential knowledge for the anatomist. The reader should refer to *Anatomy and Human Movement* (Palastanga, Field and Soames 2006) for further study.

SCIATIC NERVE AND ITS DERIVATIVES

Surface marking

The **sciatic nerve** derives its fibres from the anterior primary rami of L4 and L5 through the lumbosacral trunk, and S1, S2 and S3. It is formed **in front of piriformis** in the posterior part of the pelvis and emerges from the pelvis through the sciatic notch below piriformis and **deep to the gluteus maximus**. It is the largest peripheral nerve in the body. It runs vertically down the back of the thigh, deep to biceps **femoris**, having emerged from below piriformis approximately halfway between the greater trochanter of the femur and the ischial tuberosity. About two-thirds of the way down the thigh, it splits into its terminal branches – the **tibial** and **common peroneal nerves** (Fig. 5.1a–d). Although it is difficult to palpate the nerve directly, pressure applied over the area of its course can cause considerable discomfort to the subject.

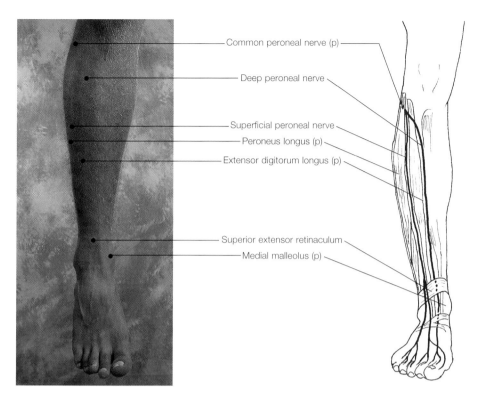

Common peroneal nerve (p)

Deep peroneal nerve

Superficial peroneal nerve
Peroneus longus (p)
Extensor digitorum longus (p)

Superior extensor retinaculum
Medial malleolus (p)

Fig. 5.1 (c), (d)
Branches of the common peroneal nerve of the right leg (anterior aspect) (p, palpable)

The tibial nerve (Fig. 5.1a,b) continues through the popliteal fossa to enter the calf **deep to gastrocnemius** and **soleus**, to lie between superficial and deep groups of muscles. It is again difficult to palpate in this region, although an unpleasant sensation can be produced if excessive pressure is applied. In the lower third of the leg the tibial nerve becomes medial to the **tendo calcaneus**, and continues to the space behind the **medial malleolus** where it is palpable. It can be traced proximally into the leg, and distally into the foot, where it almost immediately divides into the **medial** and **lateral plantar nerves**. These terminal branches soon become too deep to be palpated.

The common peroneal nerve, the lateral terminal branch of the sciatic nerve, enters the popliteal fossa. It passes down the medial side of the **tendon of biceps femoris** where it can be palpated passing behind the head of the fibula to the neck (Fig. 5.1). It then winds anteriorly around the neck of the fibula, immediately splitting into superficial and deep branches.

Palpation

With the knee semiflexed, locate the tendon of biceps femoris as it passes down to the head of the fibula,

posterolateral to the knee. Below the level of the knee joint the common peroneal nerve will be found just medial and deep to this tendon, passing behind the head of the fibula and winding forwards around the neck of the fibula (Fig. 5.1). It is easier to palpate posteriorly but more difficult anteriorly as it becomes covered by peroneus longus and tibialis anterior.

The deep peroneal nerve lies deep within the anterior compartment of the leg and is impossible to palpate until it crosses the anterior aspect of the ankle joint between the tendons of extensor hallucis longus and **extensor digitorum longus**.

First find the anterior tibial pulse on the front of the ankle joint between extensor hallucis longus and extensor digitorum longus. The nerve runs just lateral to this, but it is difficult to find as it lies deep to the **superior extensor retinaculum**.

The **superficial peroneal nerve** can be palpated passing over the anterolateral aspect of the ankle, just medial to the anterior border of the lateral malleolus. It can be traced proximally for approximately 5 cm to where it emerges from between peroneus brevis and extensor digitorum longus. Distally it can be traced on to the lateral side of the dorsum of the foot, dividing into fine terminal cutaneous branches (Fig. 5.1c,d).

SELF-ASSESSMENT QUESTIONS

Page 134

1. List the three nerve plexi which supply the lower limb.

2. From which roots does the upper plexus derive its fibres?

3. Which roots give fibres to the middle of the three plexi?

4. From which roots does the lowest plexus derive its fibres?

5. The fibres of which roots comprise the sciatic nerve?

6. In front of which muscle is the sciatic nerve formed?

7. Describe the way in which the sciatic nerve emerges from the pelvis.

8. The sciatic nerve lies deep to which muscle as it emerges from the pelvis?

9. To which muscle does this nerve lie deep as it passes down the posterior aspect of the thigh?

10. Between which two bony landmarks does the sciatic nerve pass as it emerges from the sciatic notch?

11. In which area does the sciatic nerve divide into its two terminal branches?

12. The tibial nerve enters the calf deep to which two muscles?

13. On which side of the tendocalcaneus does the posterior tibial nerve emerge?

14. In which area is the posterior tibial nerve palpable around the ankle joint?

Page 135

15. Name the two branches of the posterior tibial nerve in the foot.

16. The common peroneal nerve lies medial to which muscle in the lower part of the thigh?

17. In which area around the knee joint can the common peroneal nerve be palpated?

18. Describe how the nerve passes to the anterior compartment of the leg.

19. Name the two branches into which the common peroneal nerve splits as it enters the anterior compartment of the leg.

20. Which nerve passes across the ankle between the extensor hallucis longus and the extensor digitorum longus?

21. Does this nerve lie deep or superficial to the superior extensor retinaculum?

Please complete the labels below.

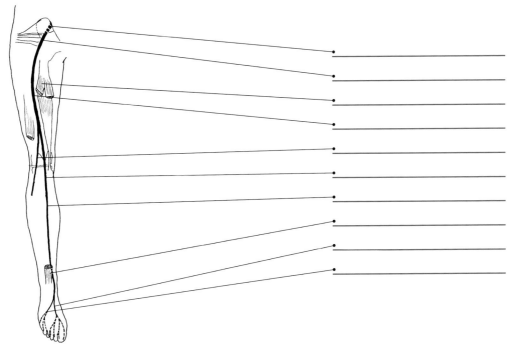

Fig. 5.1 (b) The sciatic nerve and branches in the left lower limb (posterior view)

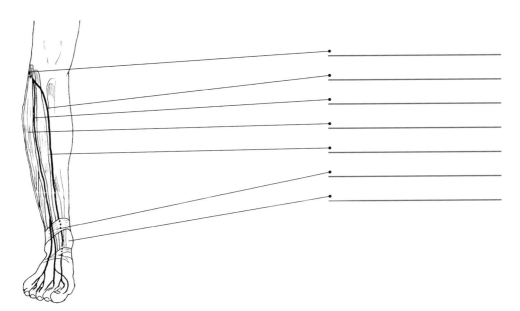

Fig. 5.1 (d) Branches of the common peroneal nerve of the right leg (anterior aspect)

22. Which nerve can be palpated as it passes over the anterior aspect of the lateral malleolus?

_____

23. Describe what happens to this nerve as it passes onto the dorsum of the foot.

_____

Chapter 6
Arteries

Contents

Femoral artery   140
Anterior and posterior tibial arteries   141
Self-assessment questions   142

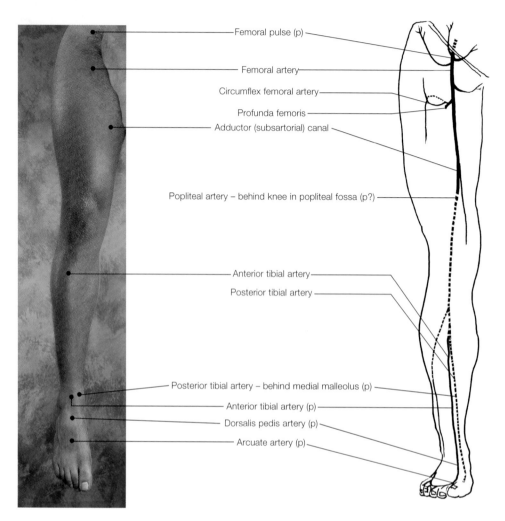

Fig. 6.1 (a), (b)
The arteries of the right lower limb (anterior aspect) (p, palpable)

Most of the large arteries are located deep within the tissues and are normally difficult to palpate.

FEMORAL ARTERY

The **pulsation** of the **femoral artery** can be palpated in the groin just below the midpoint (halfway between the anterior superior iliac spines and the pubic tubercle) of the inguinal ligament directly anterior to the head of the femur at the hip joint. Above, the vessel lies within the abdomen and below it is hidden by fascia as it lies in the femoral triangle on the proximal anteromedial aspect of the thigh. Just above the knee the femoral artery passes through the opening in adductor magnus (adductor hiatus) lying deep to the sartorius muscle in the **adductor (subsartorial) canal** to enter the popliteal fossa, becoming the **popliteal artery.** This can be palpated with deep, sensitive pressure as it crosses the back of the knee joint. Its identification is facilitated if tension of the superficial tissues is reduced by bending the knee to about 45°. Success in palpation is largely dependent on the amount of fat within the fossa and, in reality, it is extremely difficult to find. This is, therefore, a good region in which to practise the careful use of the fingers in palpation of pulses.

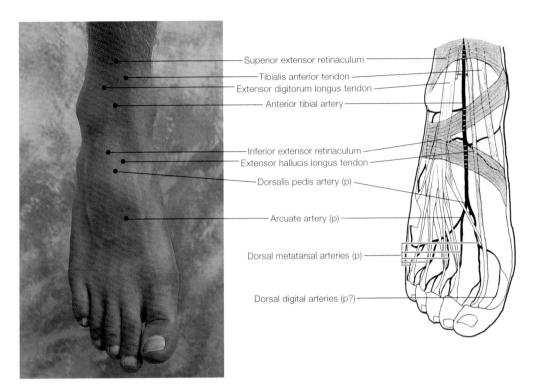

Fig. 6.1 (c), (d)
The arteries of the right foot (dorsal aspect) (p, palpable)

ANTERIOR AND POSTERIOR TIBIAL ARTERIES

As the popliteal artery enters the calf, it divides into the anterior and posterior tibial arteries. The **anterior tibial artery** passes over the main section of the interosseous membrane and below the most superior fibres (see pages 72 and 73), into the anterior compartment of the leg, deep to the anterior tibial muscles. The **posterior tibial artery** passes down the back of the leg deep to the gastrocnemius, soleus and plantaris (triceps surae).

The **anterior tibial artery** can be palpated as it crosses the anteromedial aspect of the ankle joint between the tendons of **extensor hallucis longus** and **extensor digitorum longus** where it lies medial to the deep branch of the common peroneal nerve. With careful palpation it can be traced down to the space between the first and second metatarsals where it passes into the plantar aspect of the foot between the

two bones. Beyond the **extensor retinaculum** the artery is called the **dorsalis pedis** (Fig. 6.1a–d), and is commonly the point at which the arterial supply is checked. Care must be taken not to palpate too distally, as the artery will have already passed through to the plantar aspect of the foot. In subjects with a good blood supply to the foot, the **arcuate artery**, a continuation of the dorsalis pedis on the dorsum of the metacarpals, can be palpated.

The posterior tibial artery crosses the ankle joint **behind the medial malleolus** between the tendons of flexor digitorum longus and flexor hallucis longus, medial to the posterior tibial nerve (Fig. 6.1a,b). Although it is quite clear as it crosses the ankle joint, it is difficult to trace into the medial side of the foot and the lower part of the leg.

It is important to practise finding these arterial pulses, as they give a good indication of the competence of the blood supply to the lower limb.

SELF-ASSESSMENT QUESTIONS

Page 140

1. In which area of the body may the pulsation of the femoral artery be palpated?

2. Name the gutter on the medial side of the thigh in which the artery lies.

3. Describe how the artery passes from the anterior to the posterior compartment of the thigh.

4. Through which canal does this artery pass?

5. Into which space does it pass on the posterior aspect of the knee?

6. What name is given to the artery in this space?

7. Name the muscle which lies deep to this artery.

8. List the branches into which this artery divides.

9. Describe how its anterior branch passes into the anterior compartment of the leg.

Page 141

10. Between which two tendons does the artery pass as it crosses the ankle joint?

11. Which nerve accompanies this artery?

12. Describe the course taken by the artery when it reaches the space between the first and second metatarsal bones.

13. By what name is the artery known at this point?

14. Name the artery which passes across the dorsum of the foot.

15. Describe the route of the posterior tibial artery in the posterior compartment of the leg.

16. Does the posterior tibial artery pass over or deep to the flexor retinaculum?

17. Between which tendons does this artery lie behind the ankle?

18. Which nerve accompanies this artery into the foot?

Please complete the labels below.

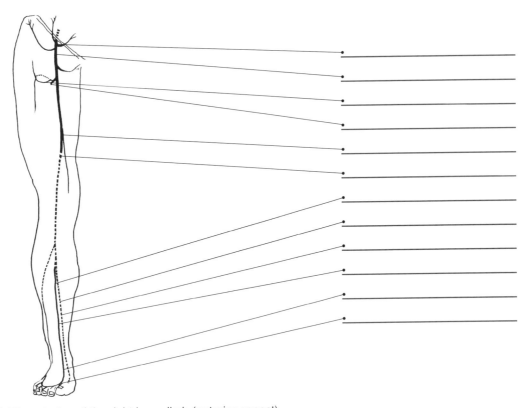

Fig. 6.1 (b) The arteries of the right lower limb (anterior aspect)

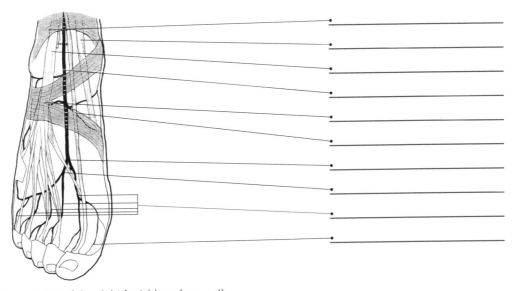

Fig. 6.1 (d) The arteries of the right foot (dorsal aspect)

Chapter 7
Veins

Contents

The deep veins   146
The superficial veins   146
    The great (long) saphenous vein   146
    The small (short) saphenous vein   147
Self-assessment questions   148

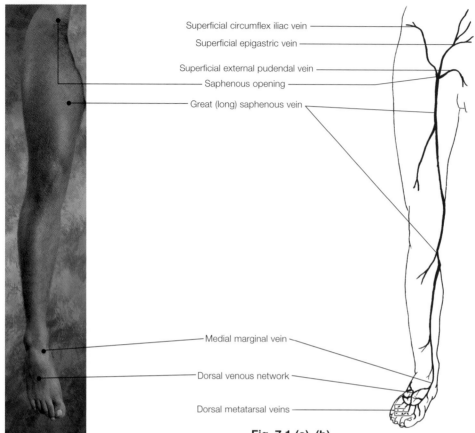

Superficial circumflex iliac vein

Superficial epigastric vein

Superficial external pudendal vein

Saphenous opening

Great (long) saphenous vein

Medial marginal vein

Dorsal venous network

Dorsal metatarsal veins

Fig. 7.1 (a), (b)
The veins of the right lower limb (anterior view)

The arrangement of veins in the lower limb is similar to that in the upper limb, there being two main systems – deep, accompanying the arteries, and superficial, contained within the superficial fascia. All veins of the lower limb possess valves, which facilitate central venous return. The valves in the communicating vessels normally only permit blood to flow from the superficial to the deep system.

THE DEEP VEINS

The smaller arteries are normally accompanied by two small veins (venae comitantes), one either side of the artery. The larger arteries are usually accompanied by a single large vein of approximately the same diameter as the artery. None of the deep veins can be palpated.

THE SUPERFICIAL VEINS

In normal subjects most veins are difficult to see or palpate, except in the distal part of the leg and on the dorsum of the foot.

With the subject standing, the **network of vessels** on the dorsum of the foot appear blue and raised. They can be palpated with little difficulty. One vein on either side of the network appears to be slightly larger than the rest; these are termed **marginal veins**.

The great (long) saphenous vein

The **great** or **long saphenous vein** (Fig. 7.1a,b) begins on the medial side of the dorsal venous network as a continuation of the **medial marginal vein**. It passes proximally in front of the medial malleolus, along the medial side of the calf and crosses the knee joint just posterior to the medial condyles of both the tibia and femur. The vein then ascends on the medial side of the thigh to join the deep system (femoral vein) after passing through the **saphenous opening** which lies below the midpoint of the inguinal ligament immediately medial to the pulsations of the femoral artery (see Fig. 6.1a,b).

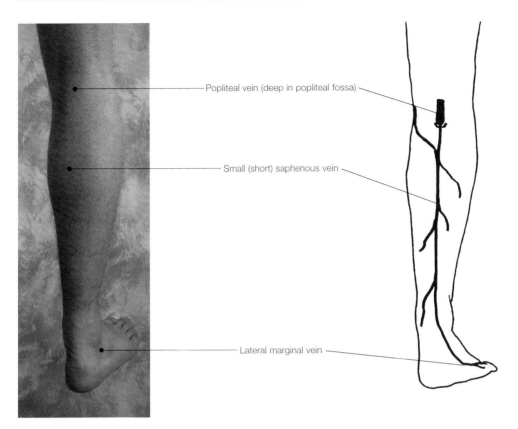

Fig. 7.1 (c), (d)
The veins of the right leg (posterior view)

Palpation

Only the lower part of the vein can normally be palpated as it lies deep within the superficial fascia. With the subject standing, find the medial marginal vein (the major vessel on the medial aspect of the dorsum of the foot). Brushing the skin surface with the finger-tips, move up to the medial malleolus. Above this level the vein can be felt passing up the medial aspect of the calf. It can often be traced posteromedial to the knee, but soon disappears as it enters the thigh. In some individuals it can be seen in the thigh as a bluish line running upwards towards the midpoint of the groin.

The small (short) saphenous vein

Beginning on the lateral side of the dorsal venous network as a continuation of the lateral marginal vein, the **small** or **short saphenous vein** passes behind the lateral malleolus and up the lateral side of the tendo

calcaneus to the posterior aspect of the calf. It pierces the deep fascia in the lower part of the popliteal fossa to join the deep popliteal vein (Fig. 7.1c,d).

Palpation

The lateral marginal vein is a little more difficult to recognize than the medial. It can be traced along the lateral side of the dorsum of the foot, but its continuation is difficult to palpate behind the lateral malleolus. That part between the lateral malleolus and the popliteal fossa is variable in its palpability; however, after a long period of standing it usually becomes quite visible and therefore easily palpable.

In some individuals, particularly the elderly, a network of vessels can be palpated on the medial side of the leg and thigh, which roughly follow the course of the great saphenous vein. Most of these join with the great saphenous vein along its length.

SELF-ASSESSMENT QUESTIONS

Page 146

1. Describe the general arrangement of the veins in the lower limb.

2. List the structures which facilitate central venous return.

3. In which direction do the communicating veins allow the blood to flow, superficial to deep or deep to superficial?

4. Name the two small veins that accompany small arteries.

5. In which areas in the lower limb are the veins most palpable or visible?

6. Name the two larger veins which run on either side of the foot.

7. Which vein drains the medial side of the foot and passes up the medial side of the lower limb?

8. Does this vein pass anterior or posterior to the medial malleolus?

9. Where does this vein cross the knee joint?

10. Which vein does it normally join in the upper part of the thigh?

11. Name the opening through which this vein passes from superficial to deep.

12. Where is this opening located?

13. Describe how this opening is formed. (fr)

14. Where can the long saphenous vein be palpated?

Page 147

15. Which vein passes up the lateral and posterior side of the leg?

16. Does this vein pass anterior or posterior to the lateral malleolus?

17. Lateral to which tendon does this vein lie?

18. Describe its arrangement in the popliteal fossa.

19. Describe a technique to facilitate the palpation of the majority of these veins.

Please complete the labels below.

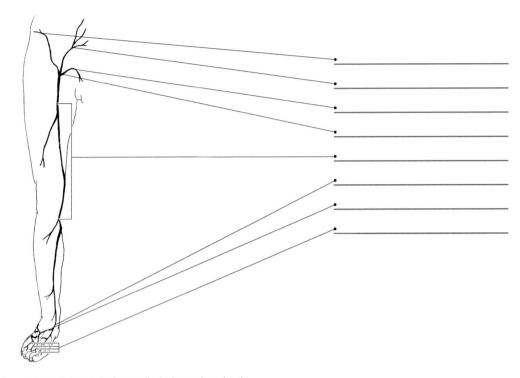

Fig. 7.1 (b) The veins of the right lower limb (anterior view)

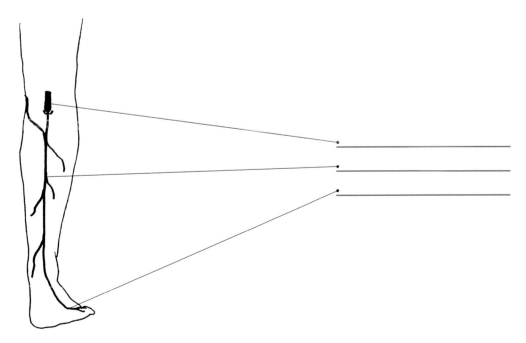

Fig. 7.1 (d) The veins of the right leg (posterior view)

References and further reading

Bayne R, Nicolson P, Horton I (eds) 1998 Counselling and Communication Skills for Medical and Health Practitioners. BPS Books, Leicestershire

Charman R (ed) 2000 Complementary Therapies for Physical Therapists. Butterworth Heinemann, Oxford

Chaitow L 2003 Palpation and Assessment Skills: Assessment and Diagnosis Through Touch, 2nd edn. Churchill Livingstone, Edinburgh

Christensen N, Jones M, Edwards I 2004 Clinical reasoning in the diagnosis and management of spinal pain. In: Boyling J, Jull G (eds) Grieve's Modern Manual Therapy: The Vertebral Column, 3rd edn. Churchill Livingstone, Edinburgh, pp 391–403

Dennis M, Jones C, Holey E 1995 Complementary medicine. In: Everett T, Dennis M, Ricketts E (eds) Physiotherapy in Mental Health: A Practical Approach. Butterworth Heinemann, Oxford, pp 252–280

Evans D 2000 The reliability of assessment parameters: accuracy and palpation techniques. In: Boyling J, Palastanga N (eds) Grieve's Modern Manual Therapy: The Vertebral Column, 2nd edn. Churchill Livingstone, Edinburgh, pp 539–546

Everett T 1997 Psychological treatment in physiotherapy practice. In French S (ed) Physiotherapy: A Psychosocial Approach, 2nd edn. Butterworth Heinemann, Oxford pp 421–432

Field E J, Harrison R J 1974 Anatomical Terms: Their Origin and Derivation. W Heffer, Cambridge

Grieve G 1986 Modern Manual Therapy of the Vertebral Column. Churchill Livingstone, Edinburgh

Guyton A C 1991 Medical Physiology, 6th edn. WB Saunders, Philadephia, pp 605–606

Hengeveld E, Banks K (eds) 2005 Maitland's Peripheral Manipulation, 4th edn. Elsevier, Edinburgh

Hinkle C 1997 Fundamentals of Anatomy and Movement: A Workbook and Guide. Mosby, St. Louis

Keogh B, Ebbs S 1984 Normal Surface Anatomy. Heinemann, London

Krieger D 1986 The Therapeutic Touch: How to use Your Hands to Help or Heal, Prentice Hall, New York

Krieger D 1993 Accepting Your Power to Heal: the Personal Practice of Therapeutic Touch. Bear, Vermont

Krieger D 1997 Therapeutic Touch: Inner Workbook. Bear, New Mexico

Krieger D 2002 Therapeutic Touch as Transpersonal Healing. Lantern Books, New York

Macrae J 1987 Therapeutic Touch: A Practical Guide. Alfred A Knoff, New York

MacWhanell 1992 Communication in physiotherapy. In: French S (ed.) Physiotherapy: A Psychosocial Approach. Butterworth Heinemann, Oxford

Magee D 1997 Orthopedic Physical Assessment, 3rd edn. WB Saunders, Philadelphia

Maitland A D 1991 Peripheral Manipulation, 3rd edn. Butterworth Heinemann, Oxford

Mason A 1985 Something to do with touch. Physiotherapy, 71: 167–169

Montague A 1978 Touching: The Human Significance of Skin, 2nd edn. Harper and Row, New York

Nathan B 1999 Touch and Emotion in Manual Therapy. Churchill Livingstone, Edinburgh

Owen Hutchinson J 2004 Health, health education and physiotherapy practice. In: French S, Sim J (eds) Physiotherapy: A Psychosocial Approach, 3rd edn. Elsevier, Edinburgh, pp 25–43

Owen Hutchinson J, Atkinson K, Orpwood J 1998 Breaking Down Barriers: Access to Further and Higher Education for Visually Impaired Students. Stanley Thornes, Gloucestershire

Palastanga N, Field D, Soames R 2006 Anatomy and Human Movement: Structure and Function, 5th edn. Butterworth Heinemann, Edinburgh

Phillips N 2004 Motor learning. In: Trew M, Everett T (eds) Human Movement: An Introductory Text, 4th edn. Churchill Livingstone, Edinburgh, pp 129–141

Poon K 1995 Touch and handling. In: Everett T, Dennis M, Ricketts E (eds) Physiotherapy in Mental Health: A Practical Approach. Butterworth Heinemann, Oxford, pp 91–101

Porter S 2002 The Anatomy Workbook. Butterworth Heinemann, Oxford

Ramsden E (ed) 1999 The Person as Patient: Psychological Perspectives for the Health Care Professional. WB Saunders, London

Sayre-Adams J, Wright S 2001 Therapeutic Touch. Churchill Livingstone, Edinburgh

Standing S (ed) 2004 Gray's Anatomy: The Anatomical Basis of Clinical Practice, 39th edn. Churchill Livingstone, Edinburgh

Stevenson C, Grieves M, Stein-Parbury 2004 Patient and Person: Empowering Interpersonal Relationships in Nursing. Elsevier, Oxford

Sunderland S 1978 Nerves and Nerve Injuries, 2nd edn. Churchill Livingstone, Edinburgh, p 355

Index

A

Abductor hallucis, 120–1
Acetabular labrum, 66
Acetabulum, 20, 66
Achilles tendon *see* Tendo calcaneus
Adductor brevis, 114
Adductor canal, 140
Adductor longus, 114–15
Adductor magnus, 114–15
Adductor tubercle *see* Femur
Ankle:
    bones, 32–5
    movements, 35
Ankle joint, 74–7
    accessory movements, 75
    line, 74, 77
Anterior cruciate ligament, 68, 71
Anterior drawer test, 71
Anterior inferior iliac spine (AIIS), 20, 21
Anterior superior iliac spine (ASIS), 17, 20–1, 66, 67, 115
Anterior tibial artery, 140, 141
Arcuate artery, 140, 141
Arteries:
    femoral artery, 140
    anterior and posterior tibial, 141

B

Biceps femoris, 30, 110, 111, 112–3
Bifurcate ligament, 82, 83, 84
Bones:
    ankle region, 32–4
    calcaneous, 34–5
    foot, 36–9
    hip region, 20–3
    knee region, 24–31
    lumbar spine and pelvis, 16–19
    palpation, 10
Braille, 3–4

C

Calcaneocuboid joint, 83, 84, 85
Calcaneofibular ligament, 37
Calcaneus, 33, 34–5, 120
    articulations, 79–84
    attachments, 118, 119
    plantar aspect, 38, 39
Calf muscles, 118–19
Circumflex femoral artery, 140
Coccygeal plexus, 134
Coccyx, 19, 22, 23

Common peroneal nerve, 30, 134, 135
Communication, non-verbal, 4–5
Consultation process, 7–8
Creams, hand, 10
Cuboid, 36, 37, 84, 85, 89
Cuboideonavicular joint, 85
Cuneiform bones, 36–7, 38, 86, 87, 88, 89
Cuneocuboid joint, 86
Cuneometatarsal joints, 86, 87, 88
Cuneonavicular joint, 86, 87

D

Deep peroneal nerve, 135
Deep popliteal vein, 147
Deep transverse metatarsal ligament, 89, 90
Deltoid ligaments, 74, 82
Dorsal calcaneocuboid ligament, 84
Dorsal digital arteries, 141
Dorsal ligaments, 85, 86, 88
Dorsal metatarsal arteries, 141
Dorsal metatarsal veins, 146
Dorsal tarsometatarsal ligaments, 87
Dorsal venous network, 146
Dorsalis pedis artery, 140, 141

E

Erector spinae (sacrospinalis), 18, 19
Examination, definition, 2
Extensor digitorum brevis, 33, 116, 117
Extensor digitorum longus, 116–17
Extensor hallucis longus, 87, 116, 117
Extensor retinaculum:
    inferior (foot), 116, 117
    superior (foot), 116, 117

F

Facet joints *see* Zygapophyseal joints
Femoral artery, 140
Femur, 24, 68
    adductor tubercle, 24, 25, 26, 30, 114
    greater trochanter, 20, 21, 22, 66
    head, 20, 21, 66
        ligament of, 66
    lateral condyle, 24, 25, 28, 29, 30
    lateral epicondyle, 24, 28

lateral supracondylar ridge, 28, 30
    lesser trochanter, 20, 21
    medial condyle, 24, 25, 26, 27, 30
    medial epicondyle, 24, 26
    medial supracondylar ridge, 26, 30
    neck, 20, 21
    patellar surface, 24, 29, 30
    upper end, 122, 123
Fibula, 24, 28–9, 31
    head, 24, 28, 29, 30, 72
    lateral malleolus *see* Lateral malleolus
    lower end, 32, 33, 34, 35, 74, 75
    styloid process, 28, 30, 68, 69
    union with tibia, 72–3
Fibular collateral ligament, 68
Foot:
    bones, 36–9
    joints, 78–93
    muscles and tendons, 116–21

G

Gastrocnemius, 118–19
    lateral head, 110, 111, 112, 113, 116, 118
    medial head, 112, 113, 118
Gluteus maximus, 110–11, 112, 113
Gluteus medius, 110–11, 112, 113
Gluteus minimus, 110–11
Gracilis, 112, 113, 114, 115
Great saphenous vein, 146–7
Great toe, 36, 37, 39, 92, 120–1
Greater sciatic notch, 22, 67
Greater trochanter, 20, 21, 22, 68

H

Hallux valgus, 37
Hammer toes, 38
Hamstrings, 112–13
Heel, 34, 36, 38
Hip bone, 20
Hip joint, 66–7
Hip region:
    bones, 20–3
    muscles, 110–13

I

Iliac crest, 16, 17, 20–1, 22, 65
Iliacus, 114, 115
Iliopsoas, 111

Iliotibial tract, 21, 112, 115, 116
Ilium, 20, 21
Inferior extensor retinaculum, 116,
    117
Inferior tibiofibular joint, 72, 73
Inguinal ligament, 16, 17
Innominate bone, 20
Intercondylar notch, 24
Intercuneiform joints, 86
Intermetatarsal joints, 78, 88–89
Interosseous ligaments:
    foot, 78, 82, 85, 86, 87, 88
    sacroiliac joint, 64–5
Interosseous membrane, lower leg,
    32, 72, 73
Interphalangeal joints, foot, 39, 78,
    90, 91, 92–3
Intertarsal joints, 78
Ischial tuberosity, 22–3, 64
Ischium, 20, 21

J
Joints:
    accessory movements, 11–12
    ankle, 74–7
    foot 78–93
    hip, 66–7
    knee, 68–71
    lumbar spine, 56–59
    palpation, 8, 11–12
    pelvis, 62
    play, 11–12
    pubic symphysis 62–3
    sacroiliac, 64–5
    swelling, 12
    tibiofibular union, 72–3

K
Knee joint, 68–71
    accessory movements, 70
    bones, 24–31
    functional anatomy, 71

L
Lateral malleolus, 24, 31, 32, 33, 34,
    35
    ankle joint, 74, 75, 76, 77
    talocalcaneal joint, 78, 79, 81
Lateral marginal vein, 147
Lateral meniscus, 25, 69
Lateral plantar nerve, 134, 135
Leg (lower):
    muscles, 116–19
Lesser trochanter, 20, 21
Ligamentum patellae, 25, 28, 68, 69,
    115

Linea aspera, 24
Long plantar ligament, 84
Long saphenous vein, 146–7
Lumbar nerve roots (L1–L5), 134
Lumbar plexus, 134
Lumbar spine, 18, 58–61
    accessory movements, 59
    joints, 58–61
Lumbar vertebrae, 18
    fifth, spine, 18, 64, 65
    laminae, 58, 59, 61
    spines, 18, 58
    transverse processes, 18
Lumbosacral plexus, 134

M
Malleolar fossa, 34, 75
Malleoli see Lateral malleolus;
        Medial malleolus
Marginal veins, 146, 147
Medial collateral ligament, 69
Medial malleolus, 31, 32, 33, 34, 35
    ankle joint, 74, 75, 76, 77
    talocalcaneal joint, 78, 79, 80, 81
    talocalcaneonavicular joint, 82, 83
Medial marginal vein, 146, 147
Medial meniscus, 25, 69, 71
Medial plantar nerve, 134, 135
Menisci, knee, 25, 69, 71
Metatarsals, 36, 37
    bases, 37, 39
    fifth, 37, 38, 39, 90
    first, 37, 38, 39, 90
    heads, 37, 38, 39
Metatarsophalangeal joints, 78,
    90–1, 92, 93
Midtarsal joint, 85
Muscle(s):
    foot, 116–17, 118–21
    hip, 110–11, 112–13
    insufficiency, 119
    lower leg, 116–17, 118–21
    palpation, 10–12
    swellings, 10–12
    thigh, 112–15, 114–15

N
Navicular, 32, 33, 36, 37, 38, 39
    articulations, 82–3, 85, 86
Nerves, 134–5
    sciatic nerve and its derivatives,
        134–5

O
Oblique popliteal ligament, 68
Obturator foramen, 20, 21

P
Palpation, 1–13
    definitions, 2
    different tissues, 10–12
    effects on patient, 6–8
    hand care, 9–10
    improving technique, 9–10
    techniques, 8–9
    touch and, 2–6
Patella, 24, 25, 28, 115
    knee joint, 68, 69, 70, 71
    movements, 27, 29, 30
Patellofemoral joint, 70, 71
Pectineus, 111, 114, 115
Pelvic girdle, 17, 20
Pelvic inlet, 16
Pelvis, 20–3
    false, 16, 20
    joints, 62–5
    movements, 23
    true, 16, 20, 21
Peroneal tubercle, 38
Peroneus brevis, 37, 38, 116, 118
Peroneus longus, 17, 18, 33, 116, 118
Peroneus tertius, 33, 117
Person–centred approach, 6
Phalanges, foot, 36, 37
    articulations, 90–3
    distal, 92
    middle, 92
    proximal, 38–9, 92, 120
Plantar aponeurosis (fascia), 38, 78,
    120, 121
Plantar calcaneocuboid ligament, 84
Plantar calcaneonavicular (spring)
    ligament, 34, 82, 83
Plantar ligaments, 84, 85, 86, 88, 90,
    92
Plantar muscles, 120–1
Plantar tarsometatarsal ligaments,
    87
Plantaris, 118
Popliteal artery, 140
Popliteal fossa, 30, 69, 112, 113, 118
Popliteal vein, 147
Popliteus, 118
Posterior cruciate ligament, 68, 71
Posterior inferior iliac spine (PIIS),
    22, 23, 64, 65
Posterior superior iliac spine (PSIS),
    21, 22, 23, 64, 65
Posterior tibial artery, 140–1
Prepatellar bursa, 25
Profunda femoris, 140
Pubic symphysis, 21, 62, 63, 64

accessory movements, 62, 65
Pubic tubercle, 17, 20, 21, 62, 66
Pubis, 16, 17, 20, 21, 62, 63

Q
Quadriceps femoris, 68, 114–15
   tendon, 25, 71, 115

R
Rectus femoris, 110, 111, 114–15

S
Sacral plexus, 134
Sacroiliac joint, 62, 64–5
   accessory movements, 64–5
Sacrospinalis (erector spinae), 18, 19
Sacrum, 16, 17, 18–19, 22
   articular tubercles, 18, 19, 22
   spinous tubercles (processes), 18,
      19, 22
Saphenous opening, 146
Saphenous veins, 146–7
Sartorius, 114, 115
Sciatic nerve, 134
Sciatic notch, greater, 22, 67
Semimembranosus, 112–13
Semitendinosus, 112–13
Shin, 24, 25, 27, 33
Short saphenous vein, 147
Small saphenous vein, 147
Soleus, 18, 118–19
Spine *see* Lumbar spine
Spinous processes, 22, 23
Spring ligament, 34, 82, 83
Subsartorial canal, 140
Subtalar (talocalcaneal) joint, 76,
   78–81
Superficial circumflex iliac vein, 146
Superficial epigastric vein, 146
Superficial external pudendal vein,
   146
Superficial peroneal nerve, 135

Superior extensor retinaculum, 116,
   117
Sustentaculum tali, 34, 35
   joints of foot, 78, 79, 80, 81, 82,
      83
   plantar aspect, 38, 39
Swellings:
   joint, 11–12
   muscle, 10–11
Symphysis pubis *see* Pubic
   symphysis

T
Talocalcaneal joint, 76, 78–81
   accessory movements, 79
Talocalcaneonavicular joint, 36,
   82–3, 84
Talonavicular ligament, 82
Talus:
   ankle, 32, 33, 34, 35
   articulations, 74–7
   foot, 36, 37, 39
Tarsal bones, 34, 36
   articulations, 78–87
Tarsometatarsal joints, 78, 87, 88
Tarsometatarsal ligaments, 87
Tendo calcaneus, 38, 116, 118, 119
Tensor fasciae latae, 110–11
Therapist–patient relationship, 7–8
Thigh muscles, 112–15
Thoracic outlet, 16
Tibia, 24, 26, 31, 68
   intercondylar eminence, 24, 25,
      31
   lateral condyle, 24, 25, 28, 29, 31
   lower end, 32, 33, 34, 35, 74, 75
   medial condyle, 24, 25, 26–7, 30,
      31
   medial malleolus *see* Medial
      malleolus
   tuberosity, 24, 25, 26
   union with fibula, 72–3

Tibial collateral ligament, 68
Tibial nerve, 134–5
Tibialis anterior, 116, 117
Tibialis posterior, 118
Tibiofibular joints:
   inferior, 72, 73
   superior, 72–3
Tibiofibular ligaments, 73, 74
Tibiofibular union, 72–3
Toes:
   bones, 36, 37, 38
   great, 36, 37, 39, 92, 120–1
   hammer, 39
   joints, 90–3
Touch, 2–6
   in clinical practice, 5–6
   expressive, 3
   instrumental, 3
   physiology, 3–4
   social significance, 4–5
Transverse tibiofibular ligament,
   73, 74
Triceps surae, 118–19
Two point discrimination test, 3

V
Veins:
   deep veins 146
   superficial veins 146
      great (long) saphenous vein
         146
      small (short) saphenous vein
         147
Venae comitantes, 146
Vertebral column, 61

W
Waist, 20–1

Z
Zygapophyseal (facet) joints:
   lumbar spine, 58, 59, 60, 61